DISCLAIMERS/LEGAL RELEASES

All patient information is within compliance with all patient privacy requirements both at the state and federal level.

CREATING A CONFIDENT SMILE

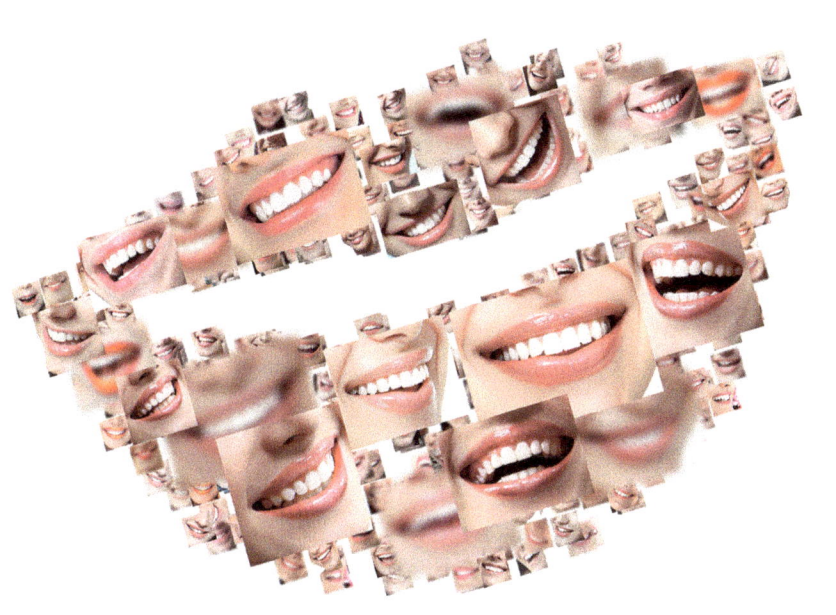

Creating a Confident Smile

Your Guide to the Smile Makeover Process

Dr. Joseph Field

PENINSULA CENTER OF
COSMETIC DENTISTRY

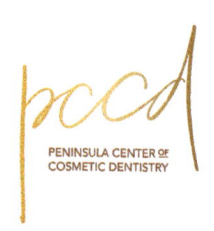

COPYRIGHT © 2025 JOSEPH FIELD
All rights reserved.

CREATING A CONFIDENT SMILE
Your Guide to the Smile Makeover Process

FIRST EDITION

ISBN   978-1-5445-4801-2 *Hardcover*
          978-1-5445-4799-2 *Paperback*
          978-1-5445-4800-5 *Ebook*

For my wife Meg, who always supports me with a smile.

Contents

Foreword 11
Introduction 13

1. The Importance of Your Smile 23
2. The Modern Dentist's Approach to Smile Makeovers .. 39
3. The Smile Design Process 55
4. The Different Types of Smile Makeover Procedures 73
5. The Smile Test Drive 95
6. Material Options and Impacts 105
7. Making You More Comfortable in the Dental Chair 123
8. The Veneer Clinical Process 135
9. Caring for Your Smile 153
10. Typical Questions and Complications 169

Conclusion 181
Acknowledgments 187
About the Author 189

Foreword

—BILL DORFMAN, D.D.S.

I first met Dr. Field in 2006. He was the president of the Alpha Omega Dental Fraternity at USC, which hosted me for a lecture on cosmetic dentistry. At that time, thanks to shows like ABC's *Extreme Makeover*, cosmetic dentistry was evolving quickly. I was fortunate to be the featured cosmetic dentist on that show, because of my expertise with cosmetic dental products like porcelain veneers and Zoom! whitening (which I invented). I have been at the forefront of Cosmetic Dentistry for decades.

Over my forty-year career as a cosmetic dentist, I've met a lot of other dentists, but Dr. Field was different. My first impression was that he was truly passionate and charismatic, but as I got to know him better, I found he was also incredibly talented. He spent a fair amount of time with me in my practice and took numerous hours of advanced continuing education units. I knew the future was bright for him, so it was not a surprise when he told me he had written this book. As a best-selling author myself, I can tell you writing a book like this while juggling a busy practice and family is extremely challenging. It is a testament to him and his dedication to dentistry and his patients.

I love the title of this book and, after almost four decades of doing cosmetic dentistry, I can tell you that this is a life-changing masterpiece. The importance of a smile is well documented, but seeing the impact cosmetic dentistry has on a person's life has been one of the greatest joys of my career. I commend Dr. Field for writing this book, sharing these stories, and for the depth of detail that will educate and empower.

Introduction

At her first consultation to talk about her smile, Sarah was in tears.

Now, I may be a dentist, but making patients cry is not the outcome I want, happy tears being the exception. I'm no Orin Scrivello, DDS from *Little Shop of Horrors*, who breaks into a happy musical number at the thought of turning his torturous dental tools on his unsuspecting patients. That image is just a myth. Since I have my own misgivings when I sit in the dental chair—I, myself, was sedated when I got my veneers—I try to do for my patients what I want done for myself in terms of communication and comfort.

No, Sarah's tears came from her embarrassment at the state of her teeth. Her prolonged, painful compensation was plain to see. She'd learned to hide her teeth with her lips while talking, which gave her a slightly odd, stiff expression when speaking. Her smile had become a kind of *Mona Lisa* image—a small uptick of the corners of the mouth that never revealed her teeth. Even smiling big enough for her pre-procedure "before" photos was hard for her to do.

The story of Sarah's smile was not unfamiliar to me. She got married young and quickly started a family. In those hectic first years, there was always something more important to attend to than fixing her teeth—potty training, school functions, family vacations, household repairs, career demands for both parents, and a mortgage. Sarah was always the last to be taken care of because she was taking care of everybody else. When Sarah turned forty and her family was more independent, she made the decision to take care of herself and get the smile makeover she'd always wanted.

That day in my office, at the very beginning of her smile transformation, Sarah said, "I can't be the person I am on the inside because of how I look on the outside." That's when she started to get emotional.

My assistant and I had seen this before. As a good dental team, we don't just treat teeth, we treat people. I stopped the meeting and got permission to give Sarah a quick hug to reassure her that everything would be okay, that I knew what we could do for her, and that she would be happy with the final result. We would get her through her smile makeover together.

After Sarah left, my assistant blurted, "I'm so excited to change that sweet woman's life!"

"I know," I said. "Her smile is going to be amazing."

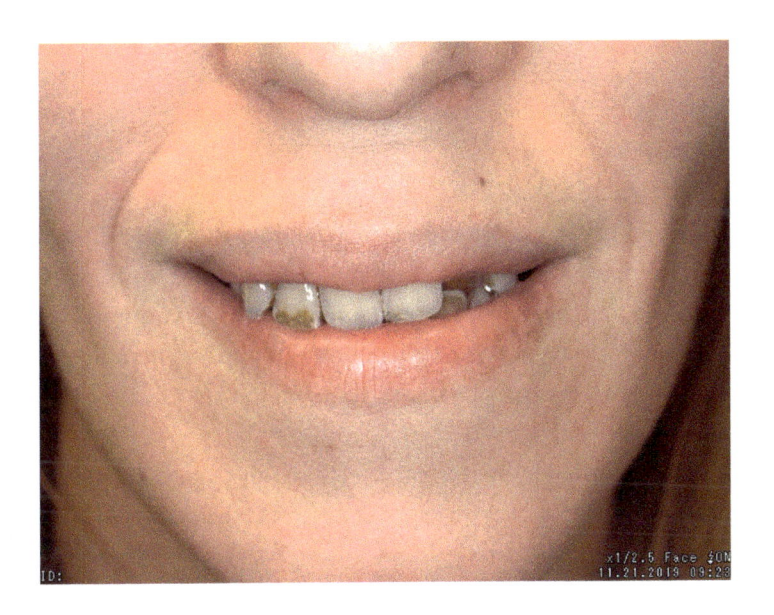

THE MISINFORMATION SURROUNDING SMILE MAKEOVERS

As a top-ranked cosmetic and reconstructive dentist in the San Francisco Bay Area practicing for more than two decades, with tens of thousands of bonded porcelain restorations under my belt, I've talked to a lot of people about their smiles. The main complaint for an incredible number of them is not the health of their teeth but the appearance of their smile. A self-conscious smile never leaves a person's mind. Every photo, every Zoom call, every social gathering, they're thinking about how everyone is looking at their imperfect teeth—and judging them. As was the case for Sarah, there exists the constant, nagging stress of trying to hide their teeth when they talk or eat, and that's no way to live life.

Humans adapt to situations, even uncomfortable or displeasurable ones, and people unhappy with their teeth are no different. They learn similar adaptations to Sarah's, to talk or smile behind their lips, or chew or bite differently to compensate for broken down teeth. They figure out how to compensate and live their lives.

But their dream is to appear on the outside the way they feel on the inside.

People often choose to live with their self-consciousness and compromises for a long time. Sometimes, it's out of misguided thinking that their teeth aren't important to prioritize. Sometimes, it's out of a general fear of the dentist's office. And occasionally, even with access to all the information out there, it's because they don't know their options.

Dentists have gotten a bad rep for centuries, and if a patient has one poor dental experience, it reinforces the perception that the dental chair equals pain. However, today's dental world is much more advanced than even just a generation ago, and we now have great options both for the aesthetics of the smile itself, and to manage the anxiety and discomfort associated with more involved procedures. Good smile design that leaves a person happy and confident has become a collaborative art with the patient, ensuring the dreaded fake-looking Chiclet smile is a thing of the past.

Fear usually comes from a lack of knowledge. Patients don't know the questions to ask of their dentists. In another twist, their regular dentist may not be able to give them good answers even if the patient does ask questions, because dentists with only standard training know little about the current advances in the world of cosmetic and reconstructive dentistry.

For a patient, getting answers from sources other than their primary dentist can be equally fraught. It should come as no surprise that social media and the internet in general are filled with dental myths and misinformation as much as cavities are filled with polymers. Quick searches using incorrect or outdated keywords only bring up pieces of the picture.

Trusting the internet for sage healthcare and cosmetic advice when someone doesn't know the real issues with their mouth or the options available is, well, not a good idea. A generalized fear of the dentist is already a big enough obstacle for most people. The American Dental Association (ADA) claims more than 70 percent of the population postpone dental care out of fear. The internet telling them to just pull all their teeth out and get dentures doesn't help matters.

The COVID-19 pandemic only fueled the problem of bad internet advice. Suddenly, everyone had a lot more time and a lot more money to pursue personal improvements. But people couldn't or wouldn't go into a dental office to talk to a provider directly. Instead, they increasingly turned to the digital world to answer their questions and tell them what to do to fix their teeth. As a result, more and more people are pursuing dental restorations (improvements to individual teeth) and reconstructions (improvements to the whole mouth) than ever before, but they are doing so with limited information at best and misinformation at worst.

A lack of knowledge about the smile design process drives a lot of poor decisions on the part of patients, such as price-shopping for a smile as they would a car. Simplifying a smile to a commodity and other misunderstandings can lead to poorly designed, managed, and executed smile makeovers. A bad makeover may result in permanent damage to the health and cosmetics of teeth, which then require even more intensive procedures to fix. Or, people just don't get the work done at all, increasing the likelihood that a full mouth reconstruction may be the only option available to them in the future.

I love information. I love learning as much as I can going into a new process or procedure so I can make the best possible choices for myself. I also love sharing the information I've learned with everyone, from colleagues to students to patients. And, at the risk of sounding immodest, I've learned a lot.

THE GOALS OF THIS GUIDE

I earned my DDS (Doctor of Dental Surgery) from the University of Southern California under the tutelage of Pascal Magne, who literally wrote the book on adhesive ceramic restorations (i.e., veneers), *Porcelain Restorations in the Anterior Dentition*, which inspired me to get into the cosmetic and reconstructive side of dentistry. I now teach at USC, and lecture and run study clubs across the country. I've completed thousands of hours of continuing education in the field and earned several national and international fellowships. My experience also includes time in my own lab, allowing me to personally oversee and work with the materials used for smile makeovers. In short, I have more knowledge about reconstructing smiles than I sometimes know what to do with. But don't worry, I've refrained from nerding out on the chemistry of various porcelains here.

While I regularly share my learning with my colleagues, students, and patients, until now I haven't had a great way of reaching the regular people across the country who need accurate, up-to-date information from a real dentist experienced in the latest cosmetic and reconstructive techniques. There's also a curious lack of any comprehensive and professional smile makeover guides for patients that I feel good about recommending. So, I wrote one myself.

The goals of this guidebook are straightforward: Show why smiles are important. Explain how a confident smile is created. Empower potential patients to seek out the smile makeover experience they want. To achieve these goals, it's important to know what to expect at all stages of the process and the possible options in terms of design, materials, and delivery of their new smile. I'll focus mostly on the veneer process, since veneers are by far the most recommended and aesthetically versatile technique used in modern cosmetic dentistry to restore and enhance a smile. Finally,

I'll go over caring for the new smile and how to handle potential complications so the smile can last well into the future.

I'll also touch on the importance of choosing a good dentist and practice that will treat each patient's unique needs. My partner dentists at the Peninsula Center for Cosmetic Dentistry (PCCD) in the Bay Area, though not directly putting pen to paper for this book, nevertheless believe and practice the same way I do. They have contributed valuable knowledge whenever a little collaboration is called for to find the best patient solution. Because of the teamwork that acts as a guiding principle at PCCD, the rest of this guide is written from a team-oriented perspective—a collective *we*. I'd also like to add that all patient names have been replaced with pseudonyms—even if the patient has given permission to use their story publicly, or already posted a testimonial on public social media—to respect their privacy.

Like for Sarah, and so many of our other patients, a confident smile isn't merely on the outside; it's an expression generated from the inside. Every person's smile is as unique as themselves. Customizing smile makeovers to each individual's needs and preferences is what we do as cosmetic and reconstructive dentists every single day. This approach should be commonplace across dental practices, but it's not. Another aim of this book is to fix that. Or at least empower anyone interested in a smile makeover to advocate for the processes and details that will result in the best smile for them, delivered in the best way possible.

Confident smiles can't be selected from a standardized menu; they have to be made to order. They're not one size fits all. A smile that looks good on one person's face may not on another's. Your new smile will ideally come from a vision you and your dentist work to realize together. And it will be just right for you.

WHAT A NEW SMILE CAN DO

One of the conversations I have with my patients outlines what their new smile can and cannot do for them. A better smile can improve a few things, not least of which is the basic healthy function of the bite, referring literally to the way the top and bottom teeth come together to take a bite, chew, and close the mouth. A good smile makeover works to enhance the look of the whole face, resulting in more confidence for the owner of that new smile. In terms of quality of life, a new smile is one of the biggest little changes a person can make for their overall physical and mental well-being.

Keep in mind, however, that dental work is not a magic external fix for internal problems. A new smile cannot heal fundamental issues with self-worth. A smile cannot make someone look like or turn them into a celebrity. It's not plastic surgery that will resculpt an entire face. It won't cure depression, and it can't mend a relationship. A dentist is not a therapist—an artist, hopefully, but not a therapist—and a smile is not a panacea. So when starting this process, I encourage people to be authentic with themselves and what they are trying to accomplish and why.

However, as seen through patient stories and testimonials in this book, a better smile often gives people a confidence boost they didn't even realize they wanted or needed on top of a mostly satisfying and stable life. And it can make people happier, simply because it makes it easier to, well, smile.

Sarah was transformed by her new smile. When she comes back into the office for regular cleanings, she holds her head higher. She no longer tries to fade into the background. Instead, she wears makeup to draw attention to her face. And she no longer hides her teeth—she fills the room with her radiance. She's a completely different person, projecting the air of confidence and security she had in her youth. In gratitude, her husband wrote us a card, noting the transformation and her newfound happiness, that read, "Thank you so much for what you did for my wife."

Sarah didn't so much change into a new person with her new smile; instead, she became the person she always knew she was. Her outside now matched her inside.

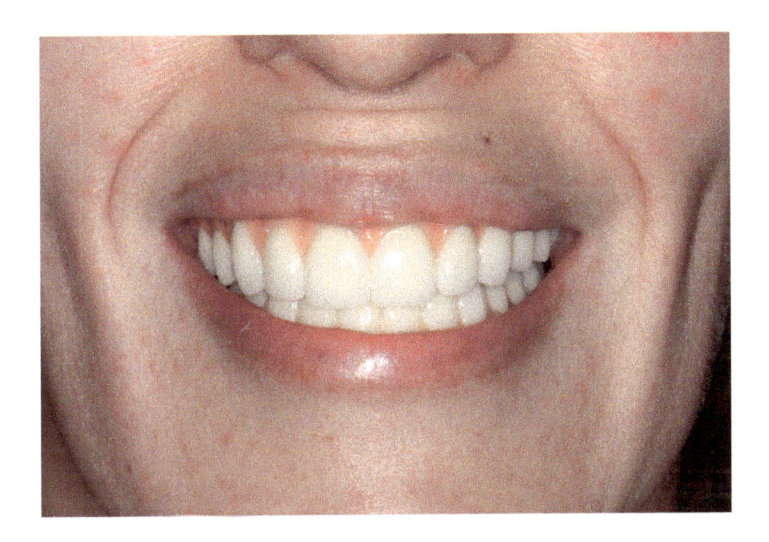

Once the onus of self-consciousness is lifted, there's less hesitation to smile. To relax. To laugh. People become much more free with their smiles, certainly more confident, and that freedom and confidence often change the way they're able to connect with others. We might have given Sarah her smile, but it was *her* smile.

To get a confident smile, you have to be confident about how your smile will be created and made a part of you. You have to feel you can take ownership of your smile makeover process, and that ownership starts before you even set foot in the office. Hopefully, the confidence that comes with the ability to make informed decisions about your health and aesthetic needs will allow you to overcome any of the challenges still holding you back from getting the smile of your dreams.

Smiles directly impact our health, self-confidence, and well-being. They dictate our comfort level in social situations. They contribute to our lifestyle choices. When we have good smiles, we feel like good guys. But if we're unhappy with our smiles, we feel like villains. And that's where we'll start the smile makeover journey, by exploring the cultural and psychological importance of the smile.

Chapter 1

The Importance of Your Smile

Mary is the daughter of a dentist, so she already knew what she should and should not be doing for her teeth. One day, she swept into our practice, expressing embarrassment about her terrible teeth and lamenting that her father would be rolling in his grave if he could see the current state of her smile. Finally, in her late fifties, she'd gotten to the breaking point and decided it was time to fix her smile.

We reassured her that it was okay to feel this way, but that we'd focus on solutions moving forward. We could reconstruct both her bite and her teeth and make her smile something to be proud of.

After she got her new smile, she was so pleased that she used her renewed sense of confidence as a springboard for other improvements to her overall health. She started exercising more, stopped smoking, and lost weight—all because she now felt more secure and happy in her body. And it all started with a smile.

Smiles are more important for people's mental and physical health than society gives them credit for, and certainly more important than the rate of trips to the dentist would imply. Since smiles impact not only our health and general well-being, but also social perceptions of our health, well-being, and even character, smile makeovers can be an emotional process.

So let's delve briefly into the psychology of the smile—why the look of a smile, especially, carries so much weight, both personally and socially. Here's why smiles matter.

WHY PEOPLE GET A SMILE MAKEOVER, AND WHY THEY DON'T

Almost a decade ago, a Fortune 50 CEO from a global tech company came into our office because of a chipped bridge. He didn't come to talk to us because his molars were ground down to the gums, or because he had no back teeth, or because of his gum disease. For him, general health and function were nowhere near as important as aesthetics and what people could see. Until the damage was visible, the state of his smile wasn't a problem for him. But now people would see this chip, and the hit to his self-confidence required a remedy. Of course, to fix the chip and keep his new bridge from breaking again, we had to fix his whole mouth to ensure the bite and teeth were healthy enough to do their jobs.

For many people, going to the dentist can invoke a lot of anxiety and fear, especially when they have neglected their teeth and now it's obvious there's a problem. The fear may originate from a sense of embarrassment because, like Mary, they've been told since childhood that they are the ones who can prevent tooth decay with proper hygiene. Failure to do so is somehow seen as a poor reflection on their values or character.

It's also interesting that some people are more willing to live with chronic tooth pain and inconvenience than go to the dentist to fix it. In the CEO's case, embarrassment about the state of his teeth had kept him out of the dentist's office for too long. However, delaying healthcare only leads to more complicated and invasive treatment procedures later on—a crown or implant, instead of a veneer, because there is little to no healthy tooth left to work with. And this delay occurs all because of the fear of the imagined mental and physical pain of the dentist's office. But once the issue becomes obvious to others, the social pressure and stigma around bad teeth force their hand.

When a person comes into the office for the first time looking for a smile makeover, often it isn't because the person is questioning their teeth; it's because someone else has. A significant other, co-worker, or friend makes a comment about the person's smile that draws attention to its flaws, and it's a powerful trigger to change things for the better. For example, one patient of mine was an elementary school teacher whose teeth had started to yellow, and whitening wasn't working anymore. Second-graders are not good at tact, but they are excellent observers of differences, and she was tired of her students asking why her teeth were so dark, what was stuck to them, or why they looked that way. You wouldn't think children could make you feel self-conscious—until they notice your teeth don't look like theirs.

Another big reason people delay care is because they are too busy taking care of other priorities. Their smile continues being shifted down the line as new emergencies come up. When people finally decide to reach out to our practice, it's because they feel their quality of life could be better with a better smile. Daily, we have conversations with patients during their first consultation appointments that boil down to, "I need to do something about my smile. It bothers me. It's something I've wanted to change for a long time. It's time to take care of myself." The decision to get a makeover is the end result of a physical and emotional burden the person has been carrying for months, even years. Decades. Finally, they can't take it anymore.

This realization doesn't come out of thin air. It's pretty uncommon for us to come across a patient who doesn't want to improve their smile. They literally see their smile every day in the mirror and on video calls, they're conscious of it when they speak face-to-face—it's just something people see and think about.

Even someone later in their life or career—who doesn't feel as much social pressure as an up-and-comer to make good impressions for promotions, networking, or socializing—can reach their own personal breaking point. Mary's story is a perfect example of this. She's mature with a well-established family and career, so why did her smile matter to her? Simply put, it had taken most of her adult life to finally give *herself* a break. One day, she looked in the mirror like she'd done countless times, and like countless times before, thought her teeth were unattractive and unhealthy. But on this day, she made a dentist appointment. Mary had thought about fixing her smile for a long time, and finally got to a place in her life where she felt she deserved to. Like a lot of patients, in her heart of hearts she wanted renewal. In the end, her makeover made a huge difference in how she felt and thought about herself.

Many of my patients are going through the transitions middle-age brings. Some are trying to level up their careers or social status, which entails self-evaluation about what they can do to improve their leadership and connections. The appearance of health and competence often factor in these conversations, and that's when smile aesthetics come into play. Some are going through big relationship changes, like marriage or divorce, that change the way they see themselves in terms of a unit with another person. Family dynamics may be shifting in other ways, like kids going off to college, which means more time to think about the next stage of their life and how they want to enter it.

Big life events have a knack for drawing people's attention to things they could improve. A restored smile becomes a physical symbol of their mental and emotional transformation. It represents a positive change in how they see themselves: new smile, new you.

Whatever specific reason brings patients into the practice, it usually boils down to one of two things: the way their smile impacts them either through their social interactions or through their health.

WHY SMILES MATTER: SOCIAL IMPACTS

Below is a photo I like to use as an example of how important the smile is. It depicts a typically handsome guy smiling at the camera, with something missing from his visage. If you're thinking, *His tooth!*, you're on the same page as the majority of viewers. But did you also notice the man's missing eyebrow?

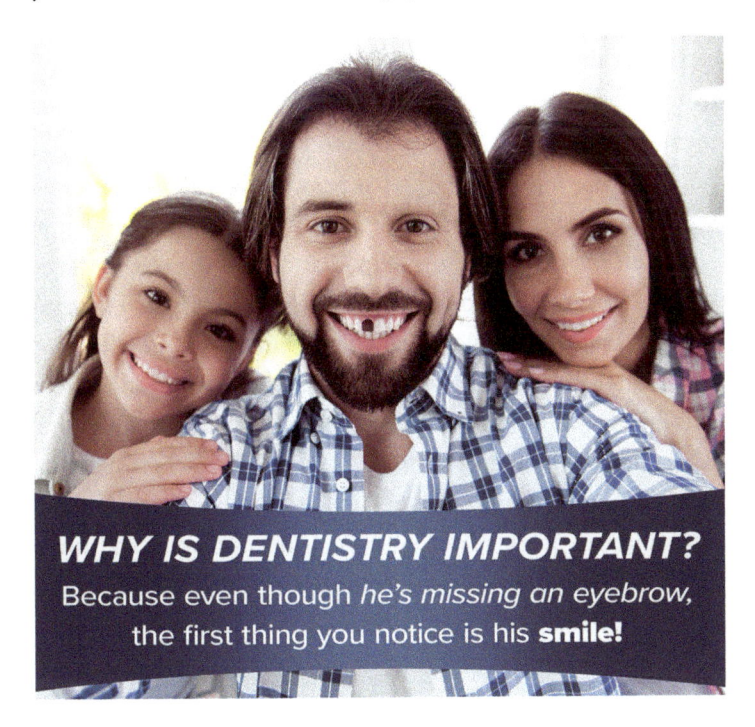

WHY IS DENTISTRY IMPORTANT?
Because even though *he's missing an eyebrow*, the first thing you notice is his **smile!**

When we look at a human face, our eyes go to the person's smile. I bet you didn't even notice the eyebrow until I mentioned it. You were likely so distracted by the missing tooth that you didn't even see the other flaws. On a scale of social importance, teeth win out over eyebrows any day of the week.

So if we pay so much attention to other people's smiles, why don't we pay attention to our own?

One of the interesting observations we've made from talking to patients over the years is the social stigma many people attach to getting their teeth fixed. When people have plastic surgery done, like breast augmentations or brow lifts, many are quick to tell all their friends and show off the work done. But when it comes to the smile, most of our cosmetic patients tell us they want the makeover to look as natural as possible so people don't know they "got their teeth fixed." They don't want to talk about it, or even admit to others they got a makeover.

To us, this reveals a layer of guilt attached to the smile and teeth that doesn't exist with other parts of the body, which makes the smile design process that much more emotionally and mentally fraught. Like with Mary, who felt her father would be mortified by her dental neglect, people seem to place an extra burden of blame on themselves for the deterioration of their teeth. Maybe because they feel they could have prevented damage, that it wasn't something they were biologically born with, like a crooked nose, or earned through legitimate experience, like a loose tummy from childbearing. Since we've been taught by our family, dentist, and educators to take care of our teeth since childhood, shame about how we "should have known better" seems to permeate all of our adult interactions with our mouths. And this shame can turn to fear of reprisal or disapproval from all quarters, especially from a dentist charged with fixing the mistakes of the past.

The smile is important because it impacts people socially—it either instills social confidence or takes it away. Everyone wants to be able to smile without reservation because they intrinsically like their smile. Everyone wants other people to think of them positively because their smile looks good. And this self-consciousness isn't a figment of the imagination. Studies show that there is real cultural psychology at work when we smile. To that point, here's a sampling of recent surveys and studies from a range of sources:

- *Huffington Post* found it only takes twenty milliseconds for your brain to register and respond to emotional expressions like the smile.[1]
- An *Association for Physiological Science* article titled "Grin and Bear It: The Influence of Manipulated Facial Expression on the Stress Response" by Kraft and Pressman found that smiling reduces stress and improves cardiovascular health.[2]
- A 2018 article by Prenger and MacDonald on the website *Dental Solutions* says our natural reaction to facial expressions is mimicry. Whether the other person gives us a smile or a frown, we tend to copy it. So, smiles really are contagious.[3]
- A *USA Today* poll shows 44 percent of those polled said the smile is the first thing they notice about another person, topping the 31 percent who said eyes.[4]

---

[1] Stephenson, Melissa. "How Smiling Can Make You Happier (in 30 Milliseconds or Less!)." *HuffPost,* December 3, 2015. https://www.huffpost.com/entry/how-smiling-can-make-you-happier-in-30-milliseconds-or-less_b_8643582.

[2] Kraft, Tara L., and Sarah D. Pressman. "Grin and Bear It: The Influence of Manipulated Facial Expression on the Stress Response." Psychological Science 23, no. 11 (November 2012): 1372–78. https://doi.org/10.1177/0956797612445312.

[3] Prenger, Margaret T. M., and Penny A. MacDonald. "Problems with Facial Mimicry Might Contribute to Emotion Recognition Impairment in Parkinson's Disease." Parkinson's Disease 2018, no. 2018:5741941 (November 11, 2018): 5741941. https://doi.org/10.1155/2018/5741941.

[4] The survey "Oral Care Love Affair: Americans Open up About Their Oral Health" was conducted via telephone during October 2010 by the Opinion Research Corporation among a nationally representative sample of 1,008 Americans ages 18 years and older.

- A survey conducted by the American Dental Association found that the smile is the number one physical feature both men and women use to evaluate attractiveness.[5]
- In a Kelton Global study, 38 percent of people polled said they would opt out of a second date with someone because of bad or misaligned teeth. Another interesting finding from that study reports that 57 percent of Americans would rather have a nice smile than clear skin.[6]
- Researchers at Swansea University found that smiles impacted perceptions of a person's health, including age and attractiveness, more than makeup.[7]
- The *Chicago Tribune* reported 74 percent believe a smile sporting discolored or broken teeth can inhibit career success.[8]
- Penn State, in "Is 'Service with a Smile' Enough? Authenticity of Positive Displays During Service Encounters," concluded that service industry employees who smile made a positive impression on their customers as opposed to those who did not.[9]
- Another study by the University of Pittsburgh, published in the journal *Perceptual and Motor Skills* in June 2012, found

---

[5] *Dentistry IQ.* "Survey Finds Smile Is 'Most Attractive' Physical Feature," February 10, 2009. https://www.dentistryiq.com/practice-management/industry/article/16371644/survey-finds-smile-is-most-attractive-physical-feature.

[6] *PR Newswire.* "First Impressions Are Everything: New Study Confirms People With Straight Teeth Are Perceived as More Successful, Smarter and Having More Dates," April 19, 2012. https://www.prnewswire.com/news-releases/first-impressions-are-everything-new-study-confirms-people-with-straight-teeth-are-perceived-as-more-successful-smarter-and-having-more-dates-148073735.html.

[7] Weston, Phoebe. "Why Simply SMILING Makes You More Attractive." Daily Mail Online, September 29, 2017. http://www.dailymail.co.uk/-/article-4933120/index.html.

[8] Wilson, Dru, and *The Colorado Springs Gazette.* "GROWNUP TEETH." *Chicago Tribune,* May 18, 1998. https://www.chicagotribune.com/news/ct-xpm-1998-05-18-9805190025-story.html.

[9] Grandey, Alicia A., Glenda M. Fisk, Anna S. Mattila, Karen J. Jansen, and Lori A. Sideman. "Is 'Service with a Smile' Enough? Authenticity of Positive Displays during Service Encounters." Organizational Behavior and Human Decision Processes 96, no. 1 (January 1, 2005): 38–55. https://doi.org/10.1016/j.obhdp.2004.08.002.

that smiling makes people look more trustworthy, and the bigger the smile the more trustworthy the models were rated.[10]
- Researchers at the universities of Leeds and Central Lancashire took pictures of people's teeth and altered their color, creating a range from bright white to yellow. The images of the whiter teeth were considered healthier and more attractive than those with yellow teeth. The perception of health even spilled over onto the overall body, as the subjects with whiter teeth were viewed as more robust.[11]

The evidence for the smile's social importance is not solely scientific. We can clearly see the cultural importance and meaning of the smile in movies and media, too. Hollywood displays in dramatic fashion that heroes have good teeth, while villains have bad ones.

For example, no matter which version of Stephen King's *It* you watch, Pennywise's smile grows more distorted, dirty, and protruding as the movie goes on to signify his growing evilness. Finally, in *Chapter Two*, the epitome of scary clowns sports so many spiny teeth in his mouth that he looks like he raided the jaws of a deep ocean fish.

In *Pirates of the Caribbean*, Jack Sparrow has horribly dirty and stained teeth until the moment the audience learns that the character is clever and fun. It's only then that we see Sparrow cleaning his teeth with a cloth, and he transitions from the role of villain to not-so-bad trickster.

---

10   Schmidt, K., R. Levenstein, and Z. Ambadar. "Intensity of Smiling and Attractiveness as Facial Signals of Trustworthiness in Women." Perceptual and Motor Skills 114, no. 3 (June 2012): 964–78. https://doi.org/10.2466/07.09.21.PMS.114.3.964-978.

11   Macrae, Fiona. "Smile! Why White Teeth Are a Sign of Good Health and Make You More Attractive." *Daily Mail Online*, August 2, 2012. https://www.dailymail.co.uk/news/article-2182380/Smile-Why-white-teeth-sign-good-health-make-attractive.html.

One of the most noticeable features of Winifred Sanderson, Bette Midler's character of the eldest witch in Disney's *Hocus Pocus*, is her two oversized front teeth.

Even when they're not in costume, celebrities are judged for their teeth. A vast majority of movie stars get work done to improve their smiles, specifically veneers. For example, John Kazinski, famous for *The Office*, admits in an interview he got his smile fixed, which, along with working out, helped take him from sitcom lead to dramatic film star. Many of our patients talk about "The Hollywood Smile" when they come to see us. Normally, it's viewed as a little *too* perfect and over the top, but it is used as a reference point for what a winning smile should look like.

The rise of remote work has taken these Hollywood considerations from the big screen to the home screen. No one wants to be known as the guy with the missing tooth or dark teeth. People often come into our practice who felt they could hide their smiles in face-to-face situations before the shift to video calls. But with the increasingly common high-def webcam close ups, that's no longer the case. Also, seeing their own faces writ large on a screen most likely highlights that their practice of hiding their teeth while they talk isn't that effective. This group of patients has become so prevalent at our practice over the last few years we even came up with a name for them: Zoomers.

As said above, a smile's *look* is often what finally brings people into a cosmetic dentist's office. A common breaking point comes when the patient realizes their smile is holding them back, whether that be in relationships, their career, or their feelings of self-worth. They realize how they look, and how they feel about how they look, matters. But of course, smiles carry more than psychological and social implications. They also directly affect our health.

WHY SMILES MATTER: HEALTH IMPACTS

Your smile is not just about its aesthetics. Healthy smiles benefit our general health, both mental and physical.

A *Psych Central* study says smiling reduces stress more than not smiling.[12] The more you smile, the more you move to a positive emotional place. The brain creates a happiness loop that encourages more positive thinking patterns. In addition, the study found smiles may strengthen the body on a cellular level. Smiling reduces the rigidity of cells, and this relaxation can help decrease the risk of stress-induced cell mutations that can lead to the development and persistence of various cancers. Yes, smiling may lengthen your lifespan and help prevent cancer!

The website *Psychology Today* explains that smiling activates neuropeptides, dopamine, endorphins, and serotonin—all of which help alleviate stress by relaxing the body and lowering heart rate and blood pressure.[13] As a bonus, dopamine is linked to neurotransmitters that increase motivation.

The Journal of Pain published a study in which participants were asked to make unhappy, neutral, and relaxed facial expressions during a treatment for pain.[14] Each group reported different levels of pain. Those who frowned said they were in more pain during the treatment than the other two groups, leading the researchers to conclude that smiling helps alleviate pain.

As a society, we're realizing that maintaining physical health goes a long way toward minimizing the amount and severity of

---

[12] *PsychCentral*. "The Importance of Smiling." Accessed January 21, 2024. https://psychcentral.com/blog/emotionally-sensitive/2018/03/the-importance-of-smiling#1.

[13] Riggio, Ronald E. "There's Magic in Your Smile" *Psychology Today*, June 25, 2012. https://www.psychologytoday.com/us/blog/cutting-edge-leadership/201206/there-s-magic-in-your-smile.

[14] Salomons, Tim V., James A. Coan, S. Matthew Hunt, Misha-Miroslav Backonja, and Richard J. Davidson. "Voluntary Facial Displays of Pain Increase Suffering in Response to Nociceptive Stimulation." *The Journal of Pain* 9, no. 5 (May 1, 2008): 443–48. https://doi.org/10.1016/j.jpain.2008.01.330.

health problems that stack up as we age. It's important to remember just how crucial good teeth are to our overall health. As time goes on, teeth and bites degrade from normal wear and tear. Teeth break down even faster if they are exposed to food and activities that aren't beneficial. Enamel can thin and stain, teeth can be in bad positions that make the bite uneven, and tooth decay and gum disease can set in.

All of these issues not only have an aesthetic component, but they also impact how well you can chew your food and what types of food you can eat, which in turn impacts digestion and how well your body can absorb nutrients. This is why women who are planning on getting pregnant are generally advised to fix any dental issues before they try for a baby. Strong, healthy teeth that function properly help to maintain—and grow—strong, healthy bodies.

A healthy mouth benefits cardiovascular health, as excessive amounts of the bacteria that causes tooth decay and gum disease can also negatively affect your heart. Some studies have even linked dental disease to a higher risk for dementia.[15] Even the way the jaws function can be connected to other bodily systems. A misaligned bite can limit room in the mouth for the tongue, thereby restricting a person's ability to breathe properly. Jaw clenching and chipped teeth can be symptoms of sleep apnea, as the body grinds the lower jaw forward to open the airway and offset lower oxygen levels during sleep.

The biggest excuse we hear for not getting a makeover is, "I know I should have come in years ago, but I just ignored it." They ignored it—until they couldn't. Aside from looks, one of the

---

[15] Sima, Richard. "Take Care of Your Teeth and Gums. Oral Health Can Affect Your Brain." *Washington Post*, September 21, 2023. https://www.washingtonpost.com/wellness/2023/09/21/teeth-gums-oral-health-dementia-alzheimers/.

biggest catalysts to bring people into the dentist's office is pain. This is generally acute, physical pain in their mouths caused by decay, deterioration, and a poor bite that taxes the muscles, joints, and ligaments of the jaw and face. But by the time physical pain becomes severe enough that it can't be ignored, the breakdown in the mouth is much more significant than simple procedures can fix.

Catching issues early is essential to avoid more intensive reconstructions that cost more and require more tooth structure removal. Remember, unlike other parts of the body, once a tooth is damaged, it does not heal or grow back.

Smiles should be more of a priority than we as a society currently give them. In terms of our social, mental, and physical welfare, our smiles matter.

YOUR SMILE MATTERS

What impacts our smile impacts us. A smile makeover doesn't just improve function and aesthetics—it can improve a person's whole attitude.

Here's the secret of a great smile: confidence. People whose smiles light up a room know their pearly whites are working for them. They are happy with how their smile looks. They are happy with how their mouth feels when they eat. They often don't understand what it means to *not* have a nice smile, because they don't have to worry about its impacts. Their smile is winning.

But those of us who have improved our smiles with restorations, from something as minor as whitening to as major as full veneers, sometimes feel we've "cheated" to get a nice smile. As if fixing our teeth cosmetically was somehow dishonest, even though we wouldn't bat an eye at fixing our teeth for health reasons.

Patients usually have one of two reactions to a compliment

on a new smile. The first group hides they've gotten work done. They say, "Thank you," and move on. The second group takes abrupt ownership of the fact their biological smile got some help, "Thanks, it's fake." Why the two extremes I'm not entirely sure, but these reactions hint at controversial cultural attitudes surrounding cosmetic procedures.

The air of social judgment and disapproval over "getting work done" on the body fills tabloids and social media daily. That seems to spill over onto the mouth and teeth, even though looks and health are intertwined when it comes to smiles. This threat of judgment means the emotion that sits behind a restored smile can be quite deep. Patients often self-deprecatingly ask us if theirs is "the worst smile" we've ever seen, which speaks to a deep self-consciousness attached to the smile as both a part of the human body and a part of human identity.

For many people, smile makeovers are a high-stakes game. As the research shows, we pay a lot of attention to the smile.[16] It's important not only in terms of what it communicates about a person's health and youth, but also their personality and character. No one wants to be compared with the metal-mouthed James Bond villain, Jaws, or become a stand-in for Dr. Stu Price a la *The Hangover*, whose missing front tooth implies a moment of cosmic irony for the dentist on the Las Vegas Strip.

We believe people shouldn't be ashamed of the state of their teeth. Life is hard, and your teeth are frontline workers. They see a lot of use. A good cosmetic dentist will be attuned to any emotional undercurrents you might express, and use compassion and collaboration to put you at ease throughout the process.

Your smile matters—physically, mentally, emotionally, and

---

16 Jaffe, Eric. "The Psychological Study of Smiling." *Association for Psychological Science (APS) Observer* 23 (February 11, 2011). https://www.psychologicalscience.org/observer/the-psychological-study-of-smiling.

socially. You can't put off fixing your smile indefinitely if you want to live the happy, healthy, vibrant life you desire. Mary didn't feel like she was held back by her old smile, but after getting her new one, she realized it was the smile she should have had for years.

Some of the fear surrounding smile makeovers comes from the misunderstanding and mythology surrounding what dentists actually do and think. Much of the information available to patients, even within dental practices, is outdated. Now that you better understand the importance of the smile, we're going to give you some pointers on what to look for in a good cosmetic dentist.

Chapter 2

The Modern Dentist's Approach to Smile Makeovers

Major makeovers represent big changes. Do-overs are difficult, and expensive. To illustrate this point, Amy found a "top-rated" cosmetic dentist in Beverly Hills through Google. Maybe trusting the celebrity address, she traveled from her home in the Bay Area to get what ended up being a full mouth reconstruction. The array of crowns and veneers was installed incorrectly, compromising her bite. She had to get most of the restorations ground off just to be comfortable. Distressed (and who wouldn't be), Amy came to us, not knowing what to do about her jaw issues and the new problems with her smile's look. With some effort, we were able to restore her proper bite and achieve the aesthetics she wanted. She told us afterward that, had she known about us, she would have saved herself the trip.

It's a lot easier to get your smile makeover done right the first time with confidence in your dental team and the process.

Even experienced clinicians who have their tech and material processes on lock find some makeovers challenging because of all the biological variants involved. Bodies sometimes don't want to cooperate with our nice, neat design plans. They throw us curve balls, and we need to know how to hit them. Or, you may want to make changes on the fly as the design gets more refined, and the dentist needs to know all the artistic tricks along the way to make the necessary tweaks without compromising health and function.

The long and short of it is: find a quality dentist you trust to get your smile right the first time, learn what that smile will cost during the initial consultation, and plan a smile makeover time frame from there. A little more time and attention on the front end of things will pay off when you leave with the smile—and health—you love.

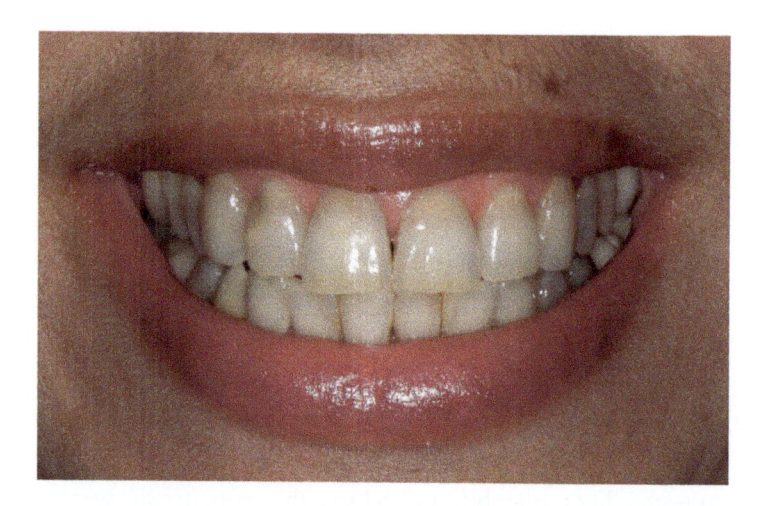

YOU GET THE SMILE YOU PAY FOR

The quality of your dentist can greatly impact your smile makeover experience, and one of the factors that can indicate quality is cost. Erin was in her twenties when she'd been inspired to get cosmetic work done after seeing the smile we'd created for her fiancé. But the COVID-19 pandemic came, and the couple elected to use a dentist closer to home in Utah rather than make the trek out to us in California. The other dentist advertised he did cosmetic dentistry, and his prices were lower than ours. And she only wanted to correct the look of her teeth, anyway. Otherwise, her teeth were healthy, functional, and in great shape.

The dentist she chose used the cosmetic procedure he knew: full crowns—on all her front teeth. But to make room for the crowns, much of her existing tooth structure was ground away. Since crowns only last a couple of decades at most, this meant the young woman now had several future crown replacements to look forward to. What's worse, she didn't like her new smile. She ended up coming back to us to fix it. We could only replace the badly designed crowns with better-looking ones. It was our only makeover option, since there wasn't enough tooth left to do veneers, the procedure she should have gotten for her particular needs.

Erin's situation is not unique. Dental work, especially cosmetic dental work, can be a big out-of-pocket expense. We sympathize with the necessity of budgeting. But the result of the cosmetic world's dependency on private pay is that patients often view dental restorations as commodities to shop for. They will call around to multiple practices, looking for the lowest price, and sometimes attempt to barter—something they'd never do for a medical procedure. Unfortunately, patients are not well-educated on the nuances of smile makeovers and don't realize ideal smiles don't come standard. Buying a smile is not like buying a car.

There are no standard makes and models. Assembly is not on a line. Parts are not interchangeable. A smile is designed to fit a particular patient's health, aesthetic, and lifestyle needs. And let's face it, a smile is part of you. It lives cooperatively with your mouth and face and bodily systems. If something goes wrong—if you find you've purchased a lemon—your body will experience the consequences.

There are some marketplace risks if cost-effectiveness is more important than the quality of the smile. Dentists just starting off may drop fees to compensate for their level of experience, and that might be okay for some people willing to assume the risk because that's the only affordable path available. But the risks are many: excessive damage to teeth; nerve damage that leads to a root canal; improper design and prep that leads to bite issues and fractures; and improper bonding and sealing that leads to decay and a shorter life for the new smile. Once a veneer or crown is done, it's done, and you have to live with it. You have to eat, after all. You can't casually scrap your mouth and replace it with a brand-new one. If something breaks down further, you have to re-do the restoration, working with the tooth structure you've got left, at considerable cost to you.

Cost cutting doesn't just extend to new dentists. Some established dentists partner with inferior ceramists, the lab technicians that construct the physical restorations, to ensure their practice is profitable. The dentist may be technically sound and deliver healthy teeth, but doesn't see the importance of a smile's aesthetics. You don't want to find a good dentist and clinic but then discover partway through the process that the ceramist uses inferior techniques and materials that lack the look and longevity you want your smile to achieve.

Cost-cutting up front often leads to more expensive outcomes for the patient later, specifically, a smile the patient hates. This last risk—a smile makeover that doesn't meet a patient's aesthetic expectations—is the most common reason we see people come into our practice when they want a redo of a prior makeover. This gains us patients, but we'd prefer the smile be done well the first time around for everyone. Therefore, knowing aesthetics often looms larger in patients' minds than health, we'd extend the idea of "you get what you pay for" to any dentists reading this book. Investing in quality lab work balances costs with patient retention and referrals.

There's a significant amount of clinical and scientific knowledge involved in producing a great smile makeover, and many dentists possess this knowledge. But where the rubber hits the road is in the fine-tuning. Like a house, you don't see the framing or foundation that's done to make the house functional. As long as those structural needs are completed properly, the house will stand. But you see and interact with the painted walls and design details every day, and if the expected amount of skill and artistry isn't reflected in those details, you're going to notice those flaws for a long time.

People shopping for plastic surgery run similar risks for negative health and cosmetic results if procedures are done by inexperienced clinicians with subpar tech and materials. While dental mistakes don't normally put people at mortal risk like plastic surgery does, a bad smile makeover does have consequences to health, livelihood, and confidence. Therefore, we suggest looking for a dentist the same way you might for a plastic surgeon, with the service provider's knowledge and skill being more important than the deal you can get on the product.

This is your body. This is your mouth. This is your health. It's a safe assumption you want changes made to an essential part of your body done right the first time.

The main objective of an effective cosmetic dentist is to idealize aesthetics while minimizing physical impact to the mouth. Prioritizing cost-cutting is only one of the factors that can hinder this main objective. A related factor to cost, a dentist's lack of training in advanced cosmetic techniques, is another hindrance. And that leads us to the myth of the crown.

THE MYTH OF THE CROWN: EASY DOES NOT MEAN BETTER

It should sound like common sense that modern dentistry leans toward the philosophy that the best work to do on teeth is the least amount of work. We want to leave as much of the original tooth structure as possible to increase a smile's longevity and maximize the options available in the future if that smile needs any more work done, either for health or cosmetic purposes. As someone who's been in the dental chair getting veneers done myself, I'm much more comfortable with the idea that the dentist leaning over me wants to use that drill lightly and doesn't get satisfaction from grinding away parts of my tooth structure.

While the sadistic dentist is definitely a myth, there are some old-school dentistry practices that may have allowed that idea to enter the popular imagination. Modern cosmetic dentistry aims to remove as little of the original tooth as possible to achieve the smile the patient wants, but many people only know about the most invasive types of makeovers. This could mean a root canal—which is only done by an endodontist to a tooth so damaged it needs drastic action to alleviate pain and keep the tooth from being pulled. But mainly, we're talking about crowns, which are often paired with root canals in people's imagination as things dentists do.

To a certain extent, the perception is right: crowns are common in dentistry practices. All dentists in dental school are trained to do them. As their name implies, crowns are a full cap that goes around the whole existing tooth above the gum line, the part of the tooth that's, not coincidentally, also called a crown. The fake crown replaces the real one. None of the original tooth is visible. To properly fit the full cap so it's not bulky in the mouth, a lot of the original tooth structure must be ground away, leaving a small tooth root for the crown to click onto, similar to how a cap clicks over a bottle top. For a tooth that already has a lot of trauma, this might be a good idea to fix decay and nerve sensitivity. The tooth is already sick, and the sick parts need replacing before they affect the root and cause more pain. Crowns are often used for these functional and health reasons. We want to be able to chew on both sides of our mouth without discomfort, after all.

But even if the original tooth is still healthy, dentists will also use crowns as a first choice restoration for cosmetic reasons, since a new cap can replace blemishes or discolorations people may not like on their existing teeth. But there are better all-around options for fixing a smile's aesthetics than replacing most of a healthy tooth with a crown, making the use of crowns for purely aesthetic reasons antiquated. The internet is no help, since the advice on its forums to get crowns is still widespread. To make it worse, some people are told by their regular dentist that their teeth are "unrestorable," implying full implants or dentures are their only option once all their teeth are pulled.

We'll discuss dentures later, but by and large, crowns are the default of many dentists, mainly because they only require standard training and are relatively easy to do. They don't take the specialized training and technical finesse that some less invasive procedures do.

Preserving the existing tooth is important. It's a general rule for many medical fields that taking things away from or opening up existing body structures results in a higher potential for that now-compromised structure having problems with breakdown, infection, or decay in the future. Think about a tire that has a nail puncture. You can patch the puncture, but the tire's lifespan has probably been decreased because it will be more prone to losing air, going flat, or having a blowout. It will need more monitoring and attention, and have a higher likelihood of needing to be replaced sooner than an unpunctured tire of the same age and wear.

As good dentists, we don't want to puncture tires we don't have to. We want to weigh the potential good health and cosmetic outcomes with those risks to functional longevity, and err on the side of caution. If we take away parts of the tooth doing a cosmetic crown, when we don't need to, years down the line when that crown may need replacement, or the tooth may need a root canal, we won't have much existing tooth to work with. In terms of available procedures, the less we have to work with, the higher the risk of having to resort to more extreme options, like pulling the tooth and putting in an implant.

In general, the more conservative we can be as dentists, the better—which means, the more tooth structure we save during a restoration, the better. Crowns may be an easier way of fixing teeth for dentists, but that doesn't make the process more effective or preferable for the patient. The more healthy tooth structure is present, the longer the life of the restoration, and the more options are available for any future restorations. Usually, this minimalist philosophy leads us toward the current favorite makeover type for cosmetic dentists and patients alike: the veneer.

THE REALITY OF THE VENEER: THE TOP CHOICE FOR SMILE MAKEOVERS

Porcelain veneers are king for cosmetic dentists. They meet all three dental goals of health, function, and artistry. Veneers are very forgiving, and very versatile to work with, so they allow you and your dentist to tweak things until they are just right. You can not only get your smile to look exactly how you want it to, but also preserve the maximum amount of healthy tooth structure in the process.

A veneer is a thin, protective layer of ceramic that is bonded to the front and biting edge of a tooth. It only requires a thin layer of the undesired or unhealthy front surface of the tooth to be removed and shaped, a process we call "prepping." The veneer is tailored to that tooth and affixed to the prepared surface, leaving the backside of the tooth mostly untouched. For prepless veneers, no grinding is done at all.

Veneers do come at a cost—a monetary one, that is. While veneers are better for the aesthetics and health of the patient's smile, those advantages require a dentist to attain additional training to do the more complex technique, as well as to have an eye for design. When we say design, we mean everything that the word *design* implies, similar to the process of customizing a piece of jewelry or the interior of a house. Color, luster, and shape are as important—if not more so—for most patients as health, function, and durability. All this requires a high level of artistry from the dentist.

Design also includes the lab portion of creating the smile, where models are turned into the material smile destined for a specific patient's mouth. The dentist is not normally the one constructing the actual porcelain restorations. That job is for the ceramist or technician in a lab the dentist partners with. In the final stages, there is close collaboration between dentist and ceramist as each veneer or restoration is given its final flourishes to make it a perfect fit. Therefore, the relationship between a dentist and lab partner is crucial to ensure the ending smile is what the patient wants and expects after seeing the smile take shape throughout the design and test drive processes.

And while we love veneers for many people who need both cosmetic and functional work done on their smiles, if the health of the tooth isn't an issue, we don't always recommend them. Sometimes the best dentistry is no dentistry. If someone can get the smile they want without veneers—say, with just some whitening and tooth straightening—let's do that instead. The main goal should be to produce not only the most confident and aesthetically pleasing smile for the patient, but also the most sustainable one—and there's nothing more sustainable than healthy biological teeth.

THE WHOLE-SELF APPROACH TO SMILE MAKEOVERS

Adhering to a conservative philosophy in terms of work done on the teeth also ensures that patients know we have the best interests of their smile at heart—their whole smile, including the lifestyle and future care that goes with it. This makes it much easier for them to trust the process if a more involved procedure is necessary to give them the confident and functional smile they want.

And this is not just the standard at our practice; the healthcare industry in general is shifting toward proactive preventative care as opposed to reactive or palliative care delivered after someone gets sick. For dentists, palliative care consists of responding to a tooth problem. If a tooth breaks, we fix it. If decay causes a cavity, we fill it. If a tooth develops nerve damage, we do a root canal. If a tooth is so far gone we can't fix it, we pull it.

In the older medical model of twenty-odd years ago, we weren't necessarily trained to look at functional or aesthetic breakdown that didn't present an immediate health problem for the patient. Dentists were merely fixers of immediate health concerns, after all. But reality shows like *Extreme Makeover*, which transformed the appearances of average people self-conscious about their bodies, started to change public perceptions in the early 2000s of what dentists could and should do. The average person saw how a smile could be completely reconstructed, not only in its health, but its appearance. And they saw in vivid close-ups the physical and emotional impact a new smile made on the people who received makeovers. It seemed a confident smile meant more to participants than any of their other alterations and cosmetic surgeries. With this revelation of the smile's importance, public demand started to shift educational dogma, and treating sick teeth became only one aspect of dentistry.

Dentists that don't challenge themselves and their training beyond the basic standard of care they're first taught can only ever remain fixers. They can't anticipate the psychological care a patient may need while going through the makeover process. They can't attain the artistry many patients now demand. And they can't reach the level of practice where they can prevent the need for restorations. Every dentist must decide if their goal is to fix teeth, or fix smiles.

A good comparison here might be an oncologist who only treats a cancer once it sets in. I wouldn't call that approach as effective as one taken by a doctor who is also trained in cancer prevention and the psychology of patients who have cancer. Medicine shouldn't just be about treating disease, but also preventing disease from establishing itself in the first place. Prevention is so much easier and inexpensive to do.

As the old saying goes, an ounce of prevention is worth a

pound of cure. The general thinking is, a tooth is "healthy" if there is no active decay, disease, or trauma causing problems. But there are other physical disease factors related to the functionality of the teeth, caused by more minor issues like tooth placement, chips, and wear. As we've seen, there are also psychological factors linked to how the teeth look in a smile, such as confidence, self-esteem, and lifestyle choices. Mary decided to take better care of her teeth once she reached a breaking point. Sarah's self-esteem increased after she took care of her teeth, which spilled over into other aspects of her demeanor and appearance. In their own ways, both women became happier after getting their new smiles.

Very few dentists are trained to handle smile designs and smile makeovers. Most view patients through the lens of function and tooth health. Stemming from their basic education in the dental field, many dentists think their primary job is to look for and cure physical disease and decay. They don't understand that there are also psychological and social components to the smile. So, even if they see a dentist regularly, the majority of people are not going to a dentist who understands their aesthetic concerns. I've had patients come in and say, "I talked to my regular dentist about improving my smile, and he told me, 'It's fine.' But my smile really bothers me, and that's why I'm here." If a patient takes the time and energy to seek out a different dentist to fix their smile, then something is far from "fine."

A good dentist will help you prevent problems and take your needs and preferences into account. Fixes won't end at stopping disease or decay, but restoring any of the damage those traumas cause. Or just giving the smile an upgrade, if that will help someone's confidence levels. It's a whole-self approach, so it's important to seek out a dentist who offers the whole package.

CHOOSING A DENTIST FOR YOUR MAKEOVER

When choosing a dentist to do your smile makeover, there are a few things you should look for:

1. Dual certification—Go with a dentist who's certified in both cosmetic and reconstructive dentistry, so they can fix both looks and function.
2. Training—Find a dentist who offers all of the modern makeover options, like porcelain veneers and implants, and has the training to deliver them well.
3. Experience—Look for a dentist with lots of experience, which means a high case count of successes, in doing the makeover you want. Years of experience may correlate to a dentist's number of cases, but not necessarily.
4. Trusted—If searching online, check out patient reviews and testimonials on several trusted review websites, such as AACD reviews (American Academy of Cosmetic Dentists), to see if former patients are happy with their smile makeover results. You could also ask family, friends, co-workers, and neighbors who've gotten makeovers if they liked their experience. Local social media groups may help here, too; just don't use them as your sole source of information.
5. Partners with a good ceramist—Check out the work the dentist's ceramic partner does in the lab. While you may not have a lot of access to that partner directly, you should have access to before and after photos. Do you like what you see? Does the artistry live up to your standards? Is there a wide range of material options and application techniques?

To help get all the information you need to make your decision, we encourage you to schedule consultations at your two or three top-choice practices. Don't feel you have to remain loyal to your current dentist. If you are offered one type of makeover, and you don't feel confident with that option, don't hesitate to get a second opinion. Some dentists won't charge for a second opinion consultation, which is another detail to check when you call for an appointment. You want the dentist you work with on your smile to check all your boxes and answer all your concerns satisfactorily. The time and resources spent will be worth it in the long run, and you'll feel more confident in the process having done some comparison.

We can't overemphasize enough the importance of having a good rapport with your dentist. If you feel doubtful going into your smile makeover journey, that lack of confidence not only hampers the successful outcome of the makeover, but also makes the process more stressful and uncomfortable. Not to get too woo-woo here, but we've seen time and again that skepticism and hesitancy on the part of the patient seem to go hand-in-hand with the weirdest things going wrong with fit, color, and durability. For example, we simply lost the final case containing the permanent veneers of one patient who still harbored a lot of fear and skepticism about the process. We've never had this happen before or since, and we'd been working so hard to answer her questions and reassure her at every point in the process. And then her smile vanished, and we had to start all over again. Whereas, patients who fully believe in us and the process have great experiences. While walking through the process in an early appointment with another patient, he stopped us and said, "Look, I'm here for a reason. I trust what you're doing. Don't worry about me." He'd tell us later to stop and focus on our work whenever we checked on how he was doing. This full-throated trust paid off for him with zero complications and perfect results.

Each dentist has their unique way of doing makeovers, ways you'll either like or dislike. So being informed is crucial to knowing your process options, empowering you to make your own health care decisions, and communicating your smile goals. Before you get set to choose your dentist, it helps to know what you want in a smile makeover process, and that starts with how your new smile takes shape.

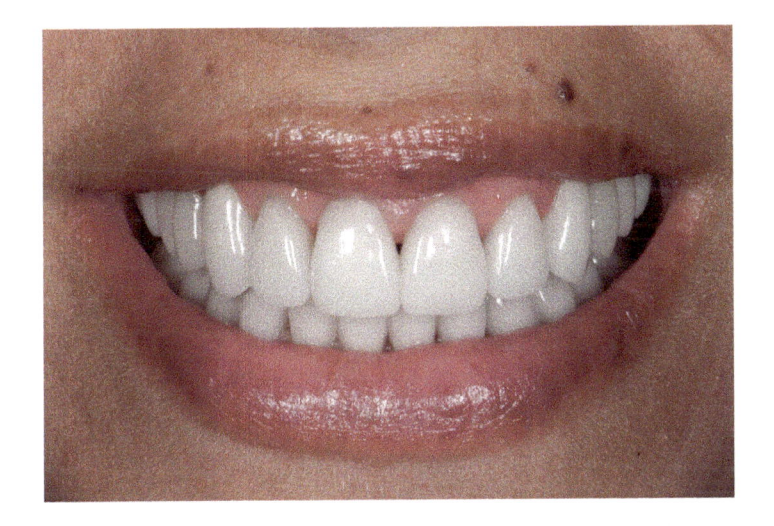

Chapter 3

The Smile Design Process

When Erin came to talk to us, she had a pretty good idea of what she wanted her new smile to look like. Her focus was on fixing her four front teeth, which were chipped and worn down. She felt that would be enough.

We took her through the full smile design process. We showed her exactly what fixing those four teeth would look like. Then, through digitized renderings of her whole face, we showed her an idealized smile based on her unique facial features and set her up with a test drive of her proposed smile—a temporary model that fit over her existing teeth. Because we had to match the restorations to existing front teeth that would remain the same, the test drive smile turned out to be darker than she wanted when she saw it in pictures. So we revised the design and did a model with ten teeth done. Consequently, we refined the design and created a model featuring ten teeth to better meet her preferences.

Her response was quick when she saw it in her mouth: "That's exactly what I want!" She had to save up more money to get the additional veneers, but she was happier doing that and waiting to get her ideal smile than getting four teeth done and being unhappy with the result.

We want each of our patients to be able to visualize what their smile will look like in their mouth and on their face. Their lips, cheeks, jaw, even the set of their features and size of their face factor into how their ideal smile looks and functions. We also want our patients to know what we're doing to their mouths and why we're doing it. We want them to feel like they are part of the process. And, most importantly, we want each person to get the confident smile that will positively resonate in their life going forward.

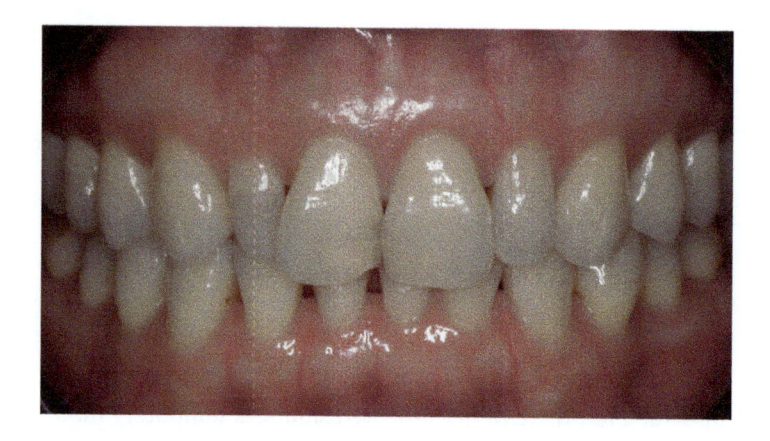

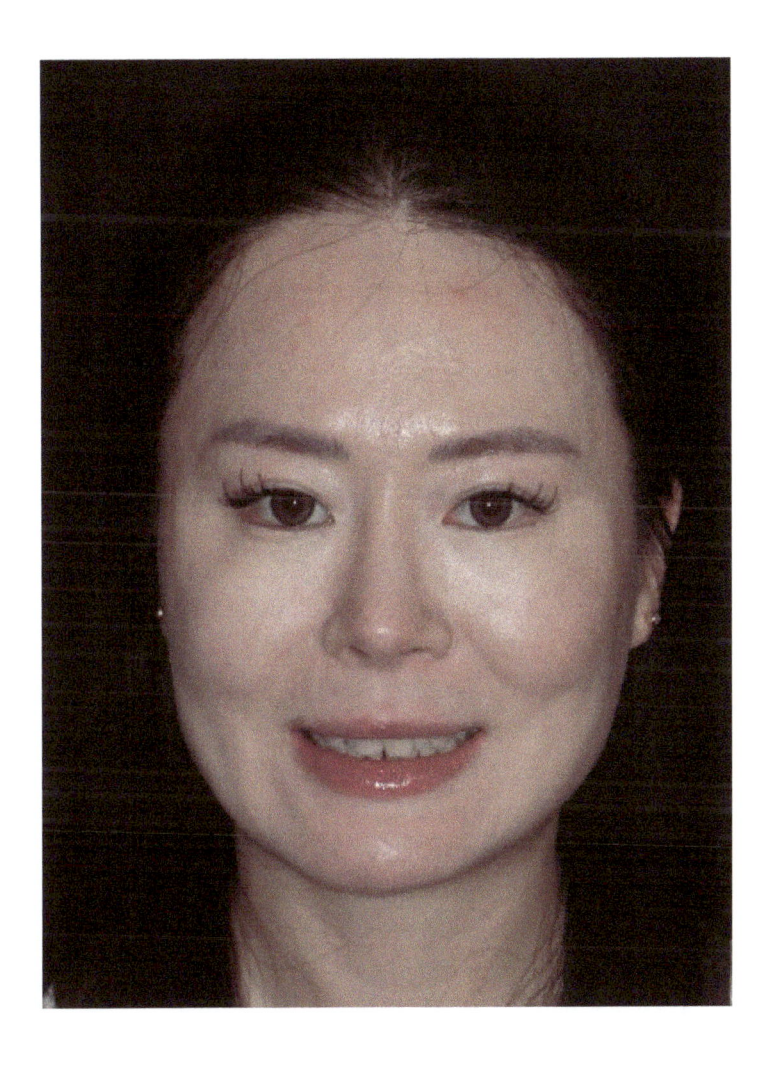

SMILE DESIGN, THE BASIC STEPS

The smile design process is a way of customizing a new smile for each individual using the most modern software and technology. The new smile is co-designed by the dentist and patient, and the patient then test drives digital and physical models of the proposed smile before they ever commit to a permanent procedure.

The power of the process is patient engagement—it grants the ability to see and try out a new smile before any work on the teeth is done.

The smile design process goes through a few steps. Since veneers account for about 80 percent of the smile designs we do, we're explaining the process of getting veneers in this book, but smile design goes through similar steps no matter the type of makeover. Those steps include:

- A consultation appointment to make sure we are a good fit. Consultations can be done in person or virtually. If we do a virtual appointment, you'll send us a picture and description of the kind of smile you're looking for prior to the appointment, and we'll do a video call to talk about the process. We'll go over all the steps, talk about comfort options during procedures, attempt to pinpoint potential complications specific to your case and plan how to mitigate them, and see if we're a good fit for you. If you want to move forward, we'll get any existing dental records, give you a quote for the full cost, get your payment information, and start designing your smile.
- A smile test drive appointment in which we create and revise a digital smile design in the office (more on this in Chapter 5).
- A prep appointment in which you get a temporary smile to try out at home for an extended period of time.
- A follow-up appointment to make any necessary adjustments to the smile design from what we learn during your time living with the temporary smile. If you have no concerns or major changes to make, this appointment can be done virtually, too.
- A delivery appointment in which we seat your permanent smile in your mouth.
- A follow-up appointment to see how your new smile is doing and to make any small changes.

We've found the whole smile design process makes for a fast, accurate, and customizable smile makeover. But the traditional smile makeover process is a bit different. The dentist will take a mold or impression of your teeth and send that to a lab technician, who will use it to make a stone model. The tech sculpts a soft wax over the top of the stone model based on arbitrary shapes and designs the technician has been taught—their version of the ideal smile using only the model teeth as a guide. Then the tech will send the wax model back to the dentist to use as a baseline for the smile design. The dentist creates a putty matrix of the tech's wax design. The patient's teeth will be prepped to receive the new smile, then the dentist will use the temporary material loaded into the putty matrix and put it over the top of the patient's prepped teeth and let that set. That's the new smile. That's how we used to do smile makeovers and how they are still done in many practices, both general and cosmetic.

The old process doesn't take advantage of all the technology that allows us to design directly within the person's mouth and face. Overlaying on models can move a design away from the uniqueness and movement of a smile that exists in a living face, making the final product look added on. And the old process does not allow for the type of patient input throughout the design process that is so valuable for creating a final product the person is happy with.

Every person's smile is unique because every *person* is unique. There are many factors that must be taken into consideration when designing a smile, and those factors go well beyond teeth.

SMILE APPEARANCE IS SUBJECTIVE

In *Something About Mary*, Cameron Diaz's character sarcastically says that she loves big teeth. The guy comically spying on her overhears this, and goes out and gets huge white square teeth, which look like a row of Chiclet candies lined up in his mouth. Of course, the joke is not the spying (which could fall flat to today's audience) but that the veneers look terrible. Completely unnatural. This scenario, of course, is poking fun at the old trend of cosmetic dentistry to default to oversized white teeth.

Not everyone can pull off big white teeth. We have patients who tell us stories of friends that got veneers done years ago, and they feel like they should be wearing sunglasses every time their friends smile. Veneers definitely shouldn't look like that.

Part of the job of the cosmetic dentist is to walk a potential patient through the smile design process and reassure them that they won't end up looking like Jim Carrey in *The Mask*, whose magical green mask exaggerates his features, not the least of which is prominent white teeth. Patients don't want hyperbole, they want a smile that fits within their face, lifestyle, and aesthetic preferences.

But what are those preferences in real life? It's common for people not to know exactly what they want when they start the smile design process. To educate patients, we discuss what the process looks like, and what factors influence the process, and then provide design options to help them envision their ideal smile. Let's take the four front teeth, for example. Typically, the front two teeth are longer than the two teeth that flank them. As dentists, we see that size difference commonly in human biology; it's a sign of youthfulness. But some people don't like that difference in length. They want all four of those front teeth to be even across the bottom. They don't want to see a gap or step up, they want the smile to be fuller and more developed. Other people are fine with the natural unevenness, and a youthful connotation is important to them. But for either type of smile, the person won't know what their preference will look like amidst the moving features of their face until they actually try it on.

Another big preference point is color. Some people expressly say they don't want the bright white "Hollywood smile," but once they see the more muted shade of natural teeth in their mouth, they change their minds and want it lighter. We turn up the brightness until we've reached the Hollywood white they thought they didn't want. Preferences range widely, and they are subjective. What looks white to us might appear too white to our patient, or not white enough—and they don't know what they really want until they see it in their own mouth.

Subjectivity extends to the entire look of the smile. Sometimes, people will bring in photos of celebrities, or a smile they found in an internet stock photo, to show us the type of smile they want. Just as they would with a hair stylist, they point to a picture and say, "I want to look like this person." We go through the design process and they get to try that smile out in their own mouths—and often they opt for something different.

The reality is, that celebrity or unknown person in the photo has a shorter nose, or fuller lips, or higher cheekbones, or a more pronounced chin. Differences in facial structure, even skin tone, factor into what smile will look ideal on what face. When Erin told us, "I want to look like Julia Roberts," we had to dig a little more to find out what that meant. What aspects of Roberts's smile did she like? If the response was, "I like the shape and color of her teeth," those are features we can play with, but also details that might not work with Erin's unique set of facial features. But if she says, "I love the way her smile fills her face," we can take that more abstract idea and dive into the conversation of design. We can talk about what we can do for her smile and to make it tie into her face—which, of course, we did. So in terms of smile design, general observations and preferences often give us more room to create.

THE GOALS FOR SMILE DESIGN

A smile design accounts for more than just appearance. Form follows function, and often the look of a smile is dependent on a smile's ability to do its biological job of eating. When we design a smile, our goal is threefold: (1) health, (2) function, and (3) aesthetics. As dentists, we prioritize goals in that order.

We don't want to just idealize the look of the teeth, we want to idealize how they do their job of chewing and supporting the structure of the jaw and face. In practice, this means taking a detailed look at how an individual's teeth and jaws work together to do the things teeth and jaws are supposed to do. This is called the bite, or how the top and bottom teeth come together to bite or chew food. Of course, the shape, size, and alignment of everyone's natural teeth and jaws vary, and a lot of times something is off, which makes the bite put pressure on the teeth unevenly. That's what causes chips, worn down teeth, and tension or pain in the temporomandibular joint (better known as TMJ).

Ultimately, the functionality of the teeth comes first, which limits what we can do aesthetically. Someone may want their front teeth to be a lot longer than what we call the "envelope of function"—in other words, their jaw movements—would allow. The models we make of their smile show them both our limitations and our opportunities.

That being said, sometimes fixing a smile doesn't impact the bone structure. It's not all about the teeth. Maybe we're going to do some gum work. We can alter the gum heights and contour the gum line to make teeth look longer or shorter. Botox can be employed to adjust lip position by calming down a lip that may jump up really high when drawn tight. In more significant cases, we do a lip repositioning surgical procedure in concert with a plastic surgeon. That's why this chapter is called the *smile* design process, not the tooth design process, since smiles are made up of so much more than teeth.

Health and function are objectively dictated by the dentist—we know what good teeth and a good bite look and feel like. As health professionals, we use all the analytical data from our CAD/CAM software and photos to make sure the smile fits and will be comfortable in each individual's mouth, customizing that functionality according to the size and shape of the mouth and existing teeth. That's what goes into the first version of the designed smile.

CAD/CAM, in brief, stands for computer-aided design and computer-aided manufacturing, respectively. It's a technology used to create, design, and then manufacture the designed product. As a process, CAD/CAM is used widely in many disciplines.

But we still consider our first design a rough draft, because until a patient has the test drive model in their mouth and walks around with it, smiles with it, it's hard for them to quantify what that new smile means for them.

In terms of that quantifying, here's a breakdown of the factors that determine a person's ideal smile:

- Face shape, size, and midline—The big picture look. How does your smile fit within the context of your whole face?
- Facial feature shape and size—How does the set of your jaw or size of your nose influence the look of the smile? We want to balance your features and ensure your smile complements them.
- Smile line—Literally, the line your smile draws across your face.
- Lip position and shape—Every person's lips will move into a different position when they smile, and tooth shape can be adjusted to work with the natural lip shape.

- Gum height (gingival architecture)—How far up the tooth does the gum line go? We can adjust this line if there's a preference.
- Tooth size—Small, large, long, or wide, we want them to look natural in the person's face and next to their other teeth.
- Tooth size and evenness—Youthful teeth tend to be shorter on the sides than in front, but some people prefer the evenness of maturity, and we always make sure new teeth have a seamless transition to the teeth that won't have work done on them.
- Tooth color—Are we going for a more natural off-white tooth color, or do we want those pearly whites? Again, we also want the new teeth to segue nicely to the old ones.
- Movement of the mouth while talking—The face is never static, cheeks and lips and jaw move all the time when you talk or laugh or smile, and we want the teeth to look good when in active conversation.
- Tooth display at rest—How much tooth shows when the mouth and face are relaxed.

All these considerations go into designing your unique smile, and it's important for your dentist to act as your guide, a sort of Jiminy Cricket through the process so you know the ramifications of each of these factors and can test out for yourself how your smile will look and work with them. Often dentists either don't have enough training to understand all these variables, or are so set in their ways they don't deviate from the smile they think is right and ignore the patient's perspective and desires. Therefore, it's important to find a dentist that is willing and able to collaborate with you and one who uses the most modern technology to do it. Otherwise, you risk going through an expensive, intense process and being disappointed with the results.

The modern smile design process is a collaboration between

the dentist and the patient. Sometimes the team expands to include spouses or loved ones, as well. We had one patient who wanted to be sedated while she got her permanent veneers, but we were concerned about getting the color the way she wanted it. So when we got to the point of trying temporary veneers on, we called her husband in to check on the color while she was asleep to get his seal of approval. Smiles, like most things, take a village to complete.

WHO HELPS TO CREATE YOUR SMILE

While a cosmetic and restorative dentist will act as the quarterback of your smile design process—the one making the calls and referrals, heading up communications, designing and constructing models of temporary smiles, delivering new smiles, and doing follow-ups—there are other players who may come into the process to lend interdisciplinary treatment planning and assistance along the way.

ROLES OUTSIDE THE PRACTICE

The roles of these players mainly apply when physical health issues need to be addressed before the new smile can be installed. In short, the foundation of the smile has to be healthy before we can design on top of it. We've ordered these specialists below, from the ones we most often work with to those we call in less frequently.

- Periodontist—They work with soft tissues in the mouth and do procedures like crown lengthening gum lifts, which take gum tissue away to make a tooth appear longer. They may also do the reverse procedure, a gum grafting, where gum tissue is added to address gum recession that may be causing sensitivity.

- Endodontist—They specialize in the nerves inside teeth, doing root canals if there's nerve damage caused by deep infections from deep cavities, abscesses, or cracked teeth. There will be a one- to two-week healing period after we fill any cavities or remove decay during prep work to see if this rare step needs to be taken before the new smile is put in.
- Orthodontist—The tooth movement specialists. They'll use braces and bands to straighten and align bite and teeth, or make room for implants.
- Oral surgeon—They take care of major bone issues, like tooth extractions, bone grafting, and installing screws for implants.
- Facial plastic surgeon—If major lip repositioning is needed as part of the smile design, we'll refer you to a plastic surgeon to alter the soft tissues of the face.

The use of these specialists is the exception, not the norm, and will differ for each individual case's needs. In contrast, the players you see inside the dental practice are involved in every smile makeover.

ROLES INSIDE THE PRACTICE

You already know about the captain inside the dental practice, but there's an entire team behind them.

- Patient liaison—They fill the role of patient advocate and help you through each step of the process, from making financial arrangements, to scheduling, to answering all your questions—or finding the person who can. Often, this is the person behind the counter when you first come in, but some practices have a designated person for this role.
- Clinical assistants—This is the team you'll see chair-side with

the dentist. They monitor records, take scans and photos, and assist with clinical procedures.
- Lab partner—The ceramist that helps create the final porcelain veneers. They'll communicate with the dentist, and sometimes the patient, to make sure the final smile design comes out just right. For our practice, that might be me, since I've gone through training to mix and make veneers.

If the dental practice you're thinking of using for your smile makeover has these players—and looks like it knows how to use them in concert—that indicates a good team.

There are a few other factors you'll also want to consider when it comes to choosing a practice, such as your budget and time. For Erin, doing ten teeth instead of four effectively doubled her budget, but the higher cost and additional time necessary to save for that cost was worth it to her after seeing her smile design. The process allowed her to prepare before anything permanent was done and, most importantly, allowed her to choose.

As another example, we've had patients who want veneers on both their top and bottom teeth but only have the budget for one set, so we'll do the top first, and then the bottom once they can afford it. These examples show how a practice can work creatively with individuals' costs, budgets, and timelines, since cosmetic dentistry is rarely covered by insurance unless there's a health problem. Even then, insurance may only cover the cheapest, most expedient option.

To sum up, the whole practice should feel warm and inviting, like it's on your side, and instill you with confidence that you'll get the smile you want the way you want.

A NOTE ON DENTAL SPECIALTIES: COSMETIC VS. RECONSTRUCTIVE

Another note on looking for a dentist: check their expertise and ensure it aligns with what your smile might need. We offer two dental specializations at our practice. The first is cosmetic. That means we can do the aesthetic aspects of dentistry, like applying veneers—strictly focusing on the way the existing teeth look. Again, to use the house metaphor, this specialty translates to the architect or interior designer.

The reconstructive expertise is something a little different and is more akin to a contractor or engineer. It concentrates on the health and function of the teeth. We can go in and do more intensive work, rebuilding bites, adding implants, and doing other procedures that replace or repair worn-out teeth and misaligned jaws.

A good cosmetic dentist should have expertise in both, as there's often some repair work to be done before cosmetics make smiles look their best and last their longest. If a patient is in their twenties or thirties, reconstructive work is less of a concern, and a purely cosmetic dentist might be enough. But if there is any doubt that the teeth or jaw will need to be realigned or repaired, going with a dual-trained dentist is recommended.

Despite our use of the metaphor of a test drive, a smile is not a new car that's assembled standard on a factory floor. A smile is an individualized and customized process. There are a lot of factors, and a lot of people involved in getting it right. That's the key to a unique smile.

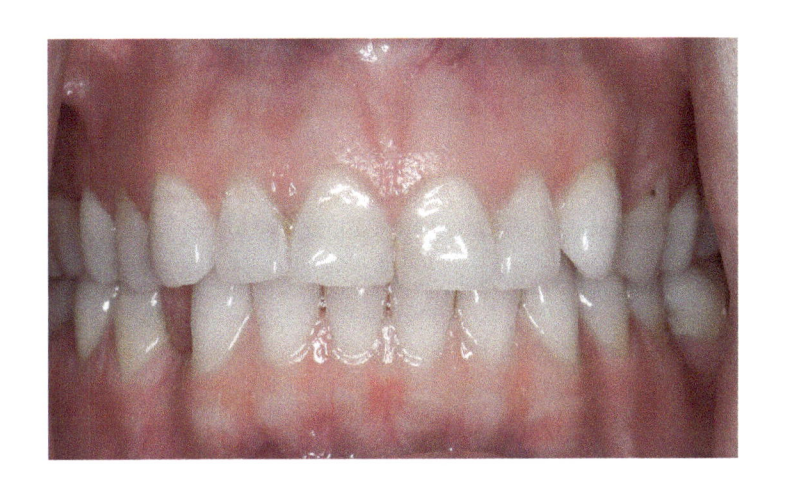

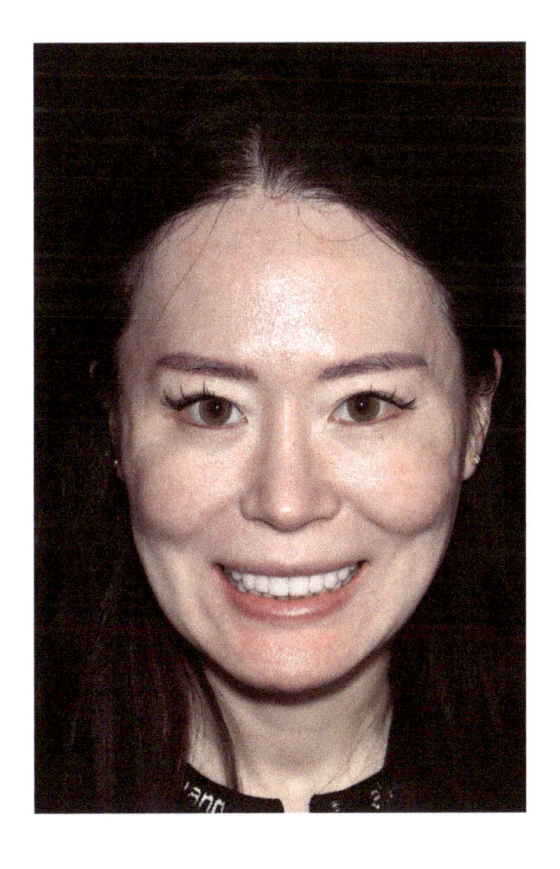

THE SMILE DESIGN PROCESS · 69

UNIQUE SMILES NEED UNIQUE DESIGNS

In the end, Erin got a smile different from the one she thought she wanted at the start. More veneers lightened the color of her whole smile and made it fuller. She was able to customize the length and shape of each tooth. While she doesn't look exactly like Julia Roberts, she got the big, broad, joyful smile that best accentuated her own features.

People often don't know what they are asking for until they see it in their own mouths. The shape of your lips, the set of your jaw, the height of your teeth, your preferences—all need to be accounted for when creating your personal smile. The confident smiles we design aren't cookie-cutter shapes. We don't select a smile "type" from a premade list of stock photos with labels like "youthful," "assertive," or "wise." Since smiles are infinitely subjective, one person's "friendly" smile may be another person's Stepford wife. A patient may think they want a natural tooth color, then see that color in their mouth with a digital image or mock-up, and decide a brighter white is what they want.

A smile is not designed to be a facelift. It won't change the existing coloring, muscle tone, or shape of a face—but it does something even better for your confidence. Our goal as cosmetic specialists is to make your smile look the best it can for you as you are. Your new smile doesn't change your face, it works with your biology to idealize your face. It shows you off to your best advantage. *I am my best*—that's the feeling of confidence we want your new smile to give you.

One size of smile does not fit all; therefore it's important to plan your smile with the right team so you can get what you want. Measure twice, cut once—that's one of our mottos. The vast majority of our time is spent in the smile design process, making sure we get everything just right so we can zero in on how you actually want your smile to look in your own mouth and face, instead of working from an abstract picture or vague idea. That way, when we go into the steps of delivering your permanent smile, the process is seamless and you have no regrets.

The smile design process gives you the power to make the best decision for you and alerts you to options you didn't know were possible. It puts you in the driver's seat. You not only help create the blueprint for your new look, but you also learn about the materials, techniques, and resources you'll need to make that happen.

Now that you know the factors that go into designing a smile, let's look at what kinds of makeovers that design might call for.

Chapter 4

The Different Types of Smile Makeover Procedures

We get all walks of life coming into our practice, sometimes quite literally.

Tim is a dog walker. When he came to us, he was already in his late sixties and had reached a point where he realized he was going to be living a lot longer and wanted his smile to live that life with him. He was a jovial and happy guy, but his smile was… not. But Tim was reluctant to talk to a dentist partly because he thought his only makeover option was dentures. His friend, also a patient of ours, talked him into checking us out. So Tim came in to explore his smile options. We told him we could do an implant-supported bridge for his top teeth and a couple crowns and implants on the bottom to fix broken and missing teeth. The combination of different restorations would create a permanent smile that would look and function like normal teeth.

When Tim heard his existing teeth could be restored and

create a smile that matched his happy spirit, he got excited. He hadn't known these restorations were available. Being able to keep what could be saved of his existing teeth and lead his normal life with his new smile meant the world to him.

Tim got his smile makeover about five years ago now. He still stops in, smiling from ear to ear. He admits he thought he could live with his old smile's problems—until we fixed his teeth and bite. Now, he says his life is better still. He commonly muses, "How did I live without this smile before?"

We want new smiles to look good, feel good, and last for a long time—and there are many ways to accomplish these goals. In this chapter, we'll show you the range of makeover options available in modern cosmetic and reconstructive dentistry. Keep in mind, a complete smile makeover may use a combination of procedures. For instance, Tim's smile was made of implants, crowns, and a bridge. Not all practices will offer the full range of makeover types, so it's important to know which procedures you find attractive and under what conditions we recommend them, so you know what to look for when selecting a practice.

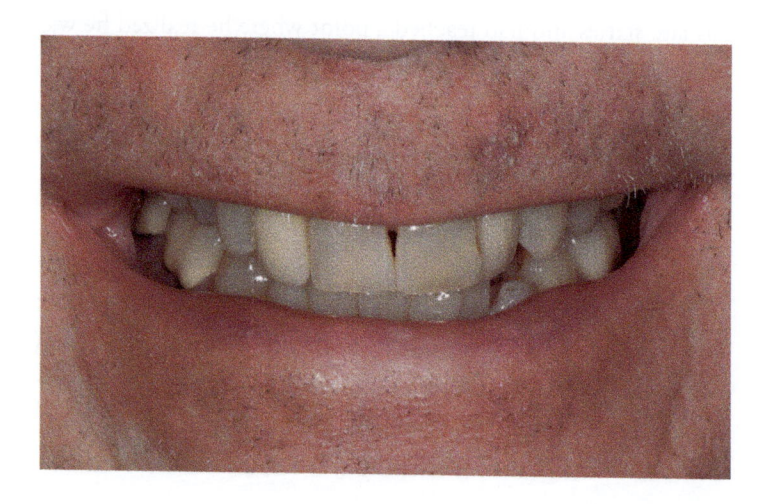

THINGS TO CONSIDER WHEN CHOOSING A SMILE MAKEOVER

When choosing your customized smile makeover, there are a few factors we consider to make sure your best interests come first. One, unsurprisingly, is patient preference. There's a world of difference between, "Make my smile look like Julia Roberts's" and, "I just want my own teeth to look better." The first request may require some major procedures and lots of fine-tuning, especially if the shape and color of the existing teeth are the opposite of what the patient wants. The second request may only call for a minimalist makeover, just some whitening or straightening, if the person is already happy with the general shape and color of their teeth.

Obviously, another factor we take into account is the health and function of the existing smile. Say the teeth have some decay or chipping, and a minimalist approach won't be enough; some restorative work also needs to be done. Often, we can combine restorative and aesthetic work, removing decay and damage and replacing it with materials that will create a healthy-looking smile.

We also want to ensure any functional issues, like an overbite or grinding habit, are taken care of with orthodontics, bite guards, or other measures so the fate of the original teeth won't befall the new smile. If you have a leak in your house, you don't just repair the soggy ceiling or floorboards, you fix the place where the leak originates. We can fix broken teeth, but if the underlying reason for the breakage isn't addressed, we'll be seeing that patient again soon to fix another busted tooth, and that ends up costing way more in terms of money, time, and health than fixing the root cause (yes, that's a dental pun!).

Two of the most common parafunctional health issues we see are clenching and grinding. Parafunctional, simply defined, refers to issues outside of the normal function of the body. For dentists, these are problems with how the jaws work. Clenching is when the jaw stiffens up and the upper and lower teeth are held tightly together. Grinding is similar, but with added movement side to side, so the teeth now also rub against each other. This constant friction wears the tooth surface down at a rapid rate, sometimes down to the gum line. Anxiety, tension, neurological or neuromuscular conditions, undiagnosed sleep apnea, and even dietary habits like chewing on bones can cause this type of unconscious, chronic jaw movement and the resulting breakdown of the tooth.

In complex cases, when teeth aren't restorable because there's too much damage or wear, we can move to more involved procedures, like bridges that use crowns and synthetic teeth to span a gap of missing teeth, or implants, which attach to tiny screws implanted into the bone of the jaw that act as roots to retain bite force and chewing functions.

Another factor may be the patient's overall health. People with diabetes or other types of preexisting health issues may not do well with makeovers that require more robust healing, as implants do, and are better served with a bridge.

There are many ways to get to the perfect smile. If a patient has crooked teeth, we may refer to an orthodontist, or the veneer process itself may provide "instant orthodontics" to those with less severe asymmetries, as we can shape the veneers in such a way that they effectively straighten the look of the teeth.

All of this boils down to one idea: the needs and wants of your smile dictate which makeover will work best for you. Like the smile design, the rest of the makeover process is customized to each unique person who steps through our doors. The following sections offer a brief rundown of the various types of smile makeover procedures available in modern dual-trained cosmetic dentistry practices.

SMILE UPGRADES

We call the following procedures *smile upgrades* because they're less involved than full smile makeovers and don't pose much risk to the integrity of the tooth structure. Procedures progress at a regular rate and stop when the smile looks right to the patient. Upgrades are strictly cosmetic, and are recommended for people who are happy with the overall shape and health of their teeth and only need small adjustments to color, positioning, or shape to get the smile they want. Because of smile upgrades' minimal interventions, they often don't require mock-ups or temporaries, and take relatively little time or money to complete. They can occur in combo with each other, or with more intensive smile makeover procedures.

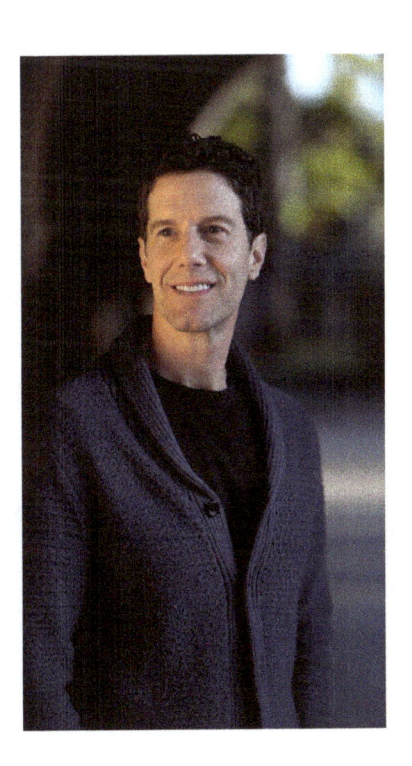

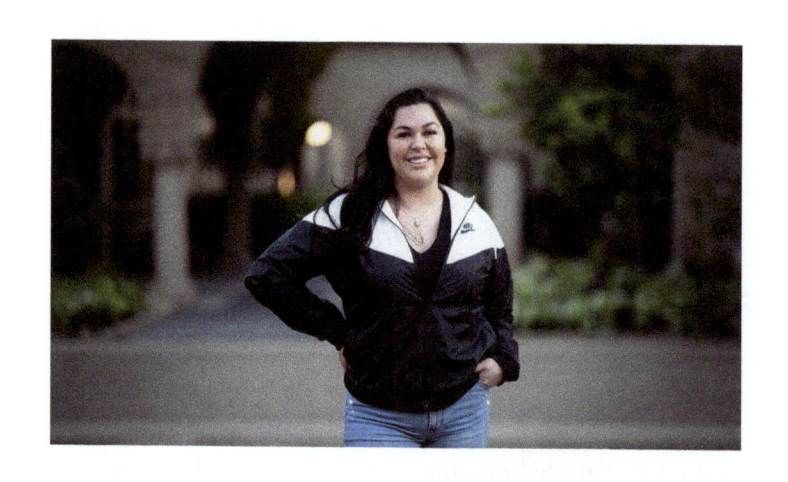

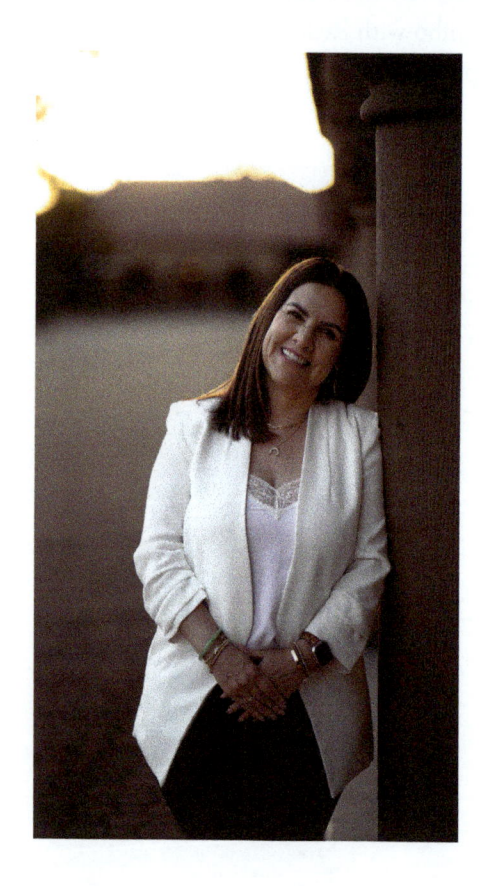

78 · CREATING A CONFIDENT SMILE

WHITENING

Whitening involves the application of good old dentist-grade hydrogen peroxide to bleach the teeth whiter and get rid of staining or darkening of the teeth. Whitening has been used in the dental industry for more than twenty-five years, and is a well-established and quick procedure with minimal impact to the teeth. Our practice offers both at-home and in-office whitening procedures, as do many others. Commonly, we do a set of four sessions at fifteen minutes each, and patients can supplement with at-home whitening trays. After each session, we'll check how the color looks, and schedule another session if desired. We do suggest going through your dentist when doing whitening, rather than buying over-the-counter options, because dentist-provided whitening is always more effective, especially in terms of time.

However, we would like to caution that whitening, out of all cosmetic procedures, is the most unpredictable in terms of success. The results of "eight shades whiter" that some commercial products advertise don't happen for the majority of people. Some teeth whiten very well and only need a couple of sessions to get to the shade the patient wants. Some teeth don't whiten at all, or minimally so, no matter how many sessions we do. We've found yellow teeth tend to whiten better than gray teeth, probably due to the nature of the staining. Gray teeth tend to result from age or staining from coffee, tea, red wine, and other dark foods like blueberries. If we get even one shade lighter, that's pretty good.

At four sessions, we're either going to have the results we want, or we're not. Whitening also reverses itself with continued life and eating habits. So, if the patient wants more dramatic results, or doesn't want to keep doing whitening treatments every three to six months, we go to veneers.

STRAIGHTENING

In modern orthodontics, teeth are generally straightened using an invisible clear aligner therapy—a thin plastic tray that goes over the teeth and slowly moves them into alignment. Clear line therapies contrast with traditional orthodontics that use brackets, wires, and bands to move the actual tooth alignment in the jaw, and sometimes the jaw itself. Cosmetic dentists often offer clear aligner therapies. If the tooth movement needs to be more drastic, like making room for an implant or correcting an overbite, braces may still be the best option, and we'll partner with an orthodontist.

SMILE CONTOURING OR TOOTH RESHAPING

If, for example, someone has really pointy canine teeth they don't like, we can do some recontouring of the teeth. Smile contouring or tooth reshaping smooths out a tooth's rough edge or takes care of a weird angle. In the canine teeth example, we'd file down the sharp cusps on the canines until they blend better with the other teeth, while still maintaining a good bite. This very minor tooth alteration doesn't have any detrimental effects on the teeth since we're staying within the outer enamel of the tooth, which is subject to natural wear anyway.

Once an upgrade calls for anything more than the above—and that includes any kind of health issue where a tooth needs to be repaired—it becomes a smile makeover.

SMILE MAKEOVERS

Smile makeovers are much more involved for you and your dental team than upgrades. They require more planning and preparation of existing tooth structure, and include some aspect of restoring healthy function to the bite and/or teeth. Often, a full makeover will involve multiple teeth. Priority is given to the front top teeth, then the front bottom teeth, both for appearance and for proper biting functions. We move next to the molars to ensure proper chewing. Because of the number of teeth and procedures involved, smile makeovers include steps for mock ups and temporary smiles and test drives (which we'll get to a little later) that give us every opportunity to make sure the permanent smile is right.

Below, we've given brief descriptions of the types of procedures you might encounter in your own smile makeover, ordered from the least to most impact on existing tooth structures. Some would be required to restore health and function, while others produce similar results and differ in their longevity, maintenance, and the way they are installed. In your initial consultation, your dentist will go over the procedures they advise for your particular needs, but a good dentist will also listen to your input on which procedures will work best for your goals and lifestyle.

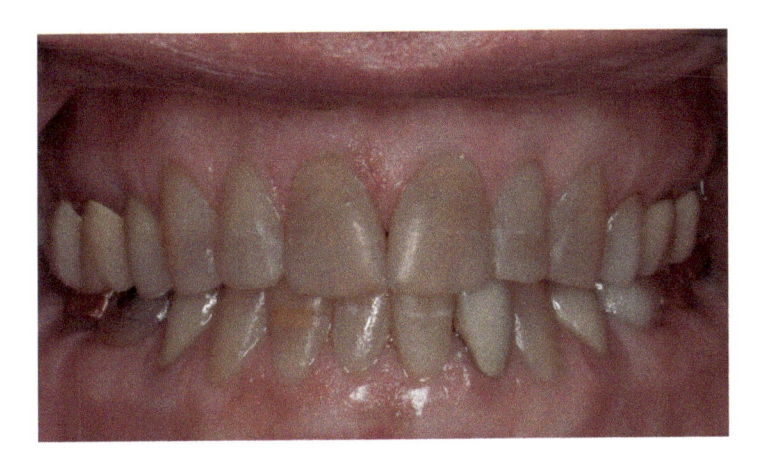

82 · CREATING A CONFIDENT SMILE

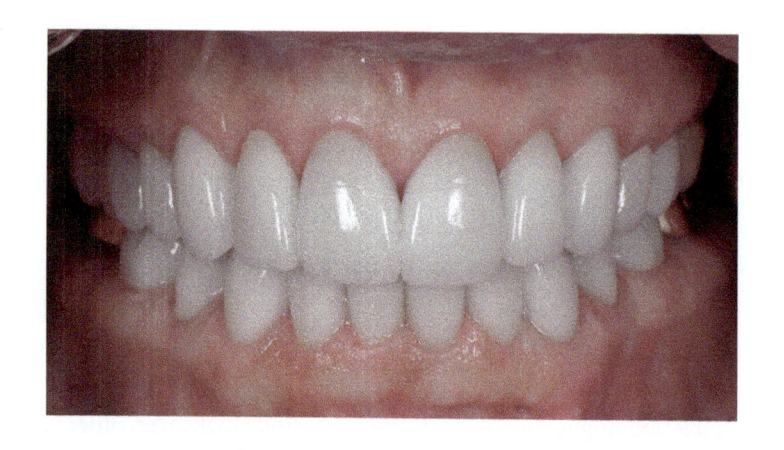

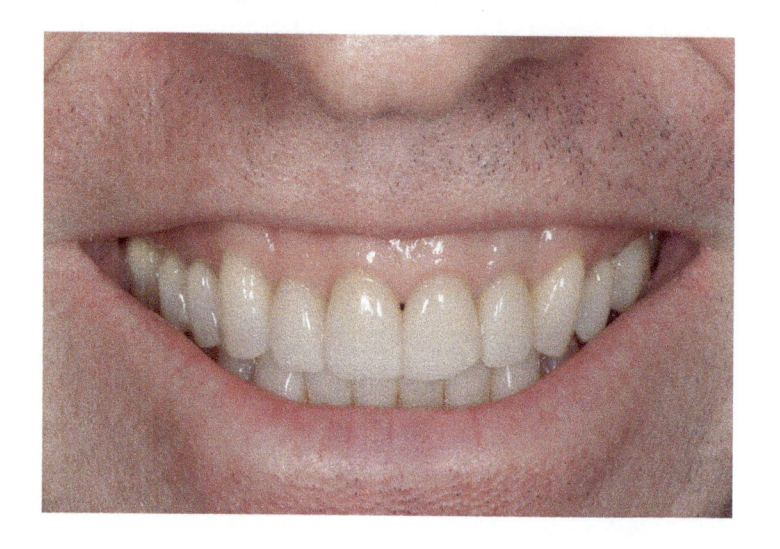

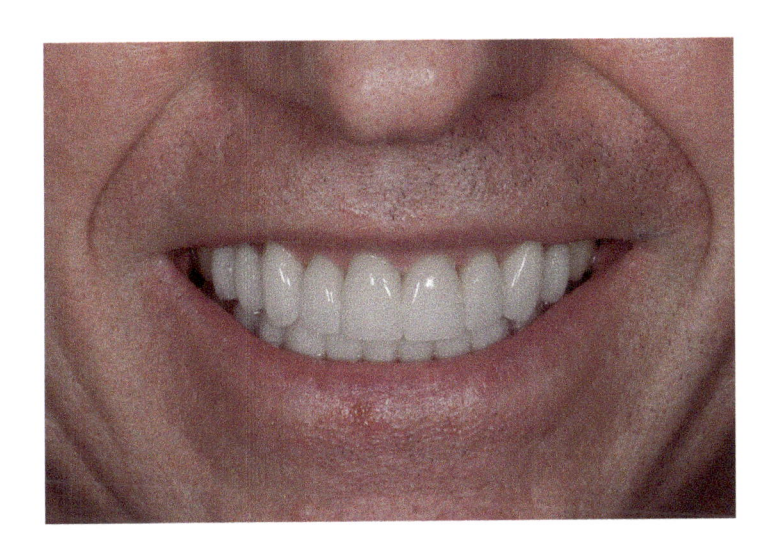

DENTAL BONDING

In dental bonding, we place a composite material, a polymer, directly over the teeth, shape it in the mouth, and cure it so that it bonds permanently to the teeth. It only takes one appointment to do this, and we can repeat the procedure easily if necessary since the tooth remains intact. Dental bonding is less expensive than true veneers, but its results are also less reliable because the bonding isn't as designed, tested, or secure as standard veneers, which means dental bonds have a higher tendency to chip and discolor and don't last as long as porcelain. The polymer also collects plaque more readily than porcelain, which can lead to more decay of the surrounding tooth. Often, bonding is used to repair a single tooth with a small chip, with restoring function quickly being the primary goal.

PREPLESS VENEERS

If a patient wants to improve the shape and color of their teeth and still get durability, all while being minimally invasive, prepless veneers may be the way to go. Prepless means there's little to no removal of the tooth structure, but a thin shell of porcelain is still bonded to the visible outer surface of the tooth.

The process has two steps. First, we make a mock-up model of the prepless veneers to test drive and finalize a smile design. Second, the ceramist uses that final design to make the permanent veneers, and we install them. Like standard veneers, the prepless ones are installed at a later appointment. However, since prepless add more material to the teeth without subtracting anything, they are only ideal for people with small teeth that have generous gaps in between them, which can absorb the extra bulk.

STANDARD VENEERS

For patients with medium or large teeth that already fit snugly together, standard veneers are the way to go. This type of makeover accounts for the vast majority of makeovers we do. It follows the same process as the prepless veneers, except the teeth are "prepped" by doing some tooth reduction and reshaping on the front face of the tooth. Porcelain is then used to fill in these spaces, applied from the gum line to just over the biting edge of the tooth. This is how we avoid the Chiclet smile, as we balance the tooth equation with both subtraction and addition to get the exact size, shape, and color the patient wants on the visible side of the tooth.

The goal is still to remove the least amount of tooth possible to get the look desired, but if more tooth structure needs to be removed because of decay or damage, the veneers will take up the slack and extend between the teeth if necessary. If gum tissue needs to be recontoured, the veneer will also account for that change. If the original teeth are dark, more tooth structure is removed to create a thicker veneer. That way, the lighter-colored veneer has the layers to better block the dark color behind it (porcelain veneers, like real teeth, have a slightly translucent quality that reflects light). And finally, if the bite is a little off, veneers can be shaped to do what we call instant orthodontics, fixing bite alignment once they are installed.

While veneers do require taking away part of the original tooth, they allow us to only take away the minimum amount needed to restore the tooth to a pristine look. The majority of the natural tooth is preserved, leading to less dental work down the line because there's less opportunity for decay or failure of the new structures. Veneers also offer the most options in terms of aesthetics, and they last a long time compared to older makeover types—up to twenty years if well cared for. Veneers are a great option for patients who want to improve aesthetics and need small functional repairs for issues such as chips, surface cracks, or staining. It's a profile that fits the majority of patients seeking makeovers.

CROWNS

If little of the original tooth structure or enamel remains because of prior dental work, or damage has progressed to the point where only the core of the tooth is still healthy, a crown may be needed to replace a tooth and restore a smile.

A crown is shaped much like a cap, and covers the entire tooth. Adding this much bulk means the existing tooth needs to be ground down substantially, leaving a small tooth nub the crown can click onto so it can use the existing healthy tooth root as an anchor point. For teeth that are cracked or already have significant decay, this level of reduction would need to happen anyway, and in these cases, a crown is the best option. We also use crowns when we have to rebuild the lingual or backside of the tooth, an area veneers don't cover. Acid erosion caused by eating too much acidic food, or cases where the patient suffered from bulimia, may expose the tooth's inner dentin, which then needs to be protected by a full crown. In general, we follow this guideline when it comes to crowns: only do them when we can't do a veneer.

IMPLANTS

Bridges were the standard of care for missing teeth before dentistry refined the implant. For most people with missing teeth, the bones of the jaws are healthy enough to support a full implant—a whole synthetic tooth structure. The process is a little involved since it requires surgery to implant a small metal peg in the jaw bone that will act as the root of the new tooth. This sounds a little scary, but it's actually less invasive than a bridge, since it takes away less existing tooth structure. Unlike a bridge, the implant also acts to replace the function, not just the aesthetics, of the missing tooth. You can bite and chew with it like a normal tooth, because it's rooted in the jaw bone. And, of course, you can floss like normal because it's not attached at the sides to other teeth, unlike a bridge.

The next part of the process is a healing period after the peg is put in place to make sure it isn't rejected. The average success rates for peg implantations are amongst the highest for medical procedures, so rejection is pretty uncommon. Then, a temporary tooth is installed for a test drive before a permanent porcelain crown is seated onto the peg, made to match the other teeth.

Implants don't impact the healthy teeth around them, and the implant is independent of its neighbors, so if something happens to it, it's just a matter of fixing the one implant. It also doesn't cause the bone recession that the more familiar tooth replacement option of dentures does. So even though the implant process is longer and takes more steps to complete than bridges do, implants are a superior solution because they are better at meeting the goals of improved appearance, health, and function.

BRIDGES

When someone is missing a tooth and implants aren't an option because of compromised jaw bones, spacing issues with the roots of other teeth, or other health factors, we do a bridge.

A bridge does just what its name implies: it bridges the gap between teeth. To do this, we have to crown the teeth on each side of the bridge to anchor the third "floating" crown of the bridge in place. The crown in the middle pushes up against the gum line but doesn't attach to it; instead, cement is used to hold it in place beside the two abutment crowns on either side, which permanently ties these three teeth together. The downside of a bridge is that damage to one tooth means the whole bridge—all three crowns—needs to be replaced. It also means we have to grind down two healthy teeth so we can form the bridge, which is always less ideal. And finally, because three teeth are now cemented together at their sides, flossing around a bridge is much more difficult and requires special tools. The additional care necessary to maintain a bridge puts the affected teeth at higher risk of decay later on.

Despite all these drawbacks, bridges still produce the aesthetic result of a full set of front teeth that most people want.

FULL MOUTH RECONSTRUCTION

It's never a pleasant experience to have a dentist tell you that all of your teeth need to be pulled out. This is what happened to a patient who came to us after consulting with a different dentist. She had a lot of old crowns and a few decayed teeth. Instead of going to the effort of saving her teeth, the first clinic she went to wanted to pull them all out and replace them with implants.

In this case, there was another option that would preserve the healthy tooth structure that remained, but it required more work and technical skill. In the end, we were able to save all of her teeth with a combination of crowns and veneers, and give her the more natural look she wanted for her smile.

Full mouth reconstructions (FMR) make some alteration to almost every tooth in the mouth. They involve a tailored combination of procedures, running the gamut from whitening to veneers to implants, that fix and replace teeth with a smile that permanently attaches. As you may imagine, this level of reconstruction is only indicated in a couple circumstances.

The first is when we're doing cosmetic work on the front teeth but there are also a lot of failing and mismatched crowns on the back teeth. If we want everything to look cohesive, prevent new decay, and restore full chewing function, we replace the old crowns at the same time we're fixing the front teeth.

The second circumstance occurs when the person has so much breakdown that their bite actually collapses as they wear down both their front and back teeth. In cases like these, there's a step we need to do before we can start on the restorations. Years', even decades' worth of clenching or misalignment, builds up tension; and this tension has to be "deprogrammed" in the muscles. This deprogramming is accomplished by using an oral appliance not coincidentally named a deprogrammer, which helps get the muscles and joints closer to the position we'll want them in permanently. In the mouth, the deprogrammer only allows the front teeth to make contact. By giving the bite a break from its daily grind, the deprogrammer relaxes and repositions the jaw. It's a little like retraining the body as someone would through exercise, getting those parts used to the idea of a new position. Bodies that are warmed up and loose are less inclined to experience painful aches and pains after the exercise, and jaws are no different. Retraining the muscles also reduces the risk of chips caused by a tension-filled bite later on.

After doing the pre-procedures that realign and shift the muscles and joints, which are steps toward the permanent smile installation, we can use an orthotic device, another oral appliance that's designed to take the stress off the jaw joints and alleviate muscle strain. Coupled with hot and cold therapy, massage, and other methods that help sore muscles and joints, a majority of joint discomfort caused by the initial realignment goes away.

Usually, FMR patients' chief complaint is the look of their front teeth, like our tech CEO. But if we don't address the wear in the back as well, any repairs we do to the front won't last long. In these cases, we need to fix the bite by "opening the vertical dimension," which sounds like something you might hear walking down Haight-Ashbury, but means we have to make the teeth a little taller with crowns to "open" the bite back to the correct position.

Another type of FMR is recommended for people who are already in dentures, or who only have a few teeth left that have reached the point of no return. For these patients, we'll then do a combination of implants and bridges. For instance, we'll place anywhere from four to eight implants in the upper jaw and create a single bridge that attaches to those implants. The whole array becomes a new, permanent smile.

And to dispel another myth, implant restorations are not just for the elderly or those with poor dental hygiene. We have a forty-year-old patient who, due in large part to unfortunate genetics and in small part to neglecting herself to prioritize her family, found herself with a mouthful of loose and infected teeth. The best option for her to get a functional smile back was to replace all her teeth with implants, set in her still-healthy jaw bones. Since she was so young, the three- to five-year lifespan of dentures and their tendency to cause bone loss was an unacceptable option.

DENTURES

Dentures *are* still a smile makeover option to replace some of the appearance and function of a smile, mainly because they are relatively inexpensive, but they are the worst way to go for a few reasons. One, your bite force is dramatically reduced with dentures, which impacts how well you can bite and chew. Two, dentures cover up taste buds on the roof of your mouth, so food will never taste the same again. Three, you lose the nerves at the root of your teeth, so sensations like hot or cold are compromised and foods like ice cream and coffee will feel and taste different. Four, pulling teeth out takes away bone in your jaws, which eventually causes more and more bone recession. Dentures have to be remade every three to five years because of these bone changes in the mouth. Eventually, the mouth gets to the point where there's no bone left for the dentures to attach to, and a dental glue like Poly Grip is the only thing holding the smile in place. There's a reason why the global dental adhesive and sealant market is estimated at over three billion dollars—the end result of dentures is a lot of glue.

In addition to their health drawbacks, they present a few other problems, as well. They are removable, and can fall out at inconvenient times, not to mention they can be snagged by the dog or passing toddler. They're also easy to identify as restorations because they are plastic, which is not the case with an implant or bridge, and certainly not with veneers. Implants and bridges are a huge upgrade from dentures in terms of our three main goals of a makeover, and vastly preferred for full mouth reconstructions. If a patient already has dentures, we'll often transition to the use of implants if that's a viable option, or possibly use surgical interventions—a bone graft or ridge augmentation—to reinforce the jaws so they can hold an implant.

And with that, we conclude the current tooth restoration makeover options. But since smiles always account for more than teeth, there are a few other things we can do to form a complete smile.

ADDITIONAL SMILE MAKEOVER OPTIONS

When doing smile makeovers, small and large, there are a few procedures that can be done to address both health and aesthetic issues with the soft tissues of the smile—the muscles, lips, and gums—that also contribute to a complete smile. The inclusion of these procedures in a full smile makeover is one of the reasons we like the term *smile makeover* to talk about the complete process, as opposed to the term *restoration*, which only refers to the tooth structure. The procedures listed below may fall within the skillset of the cosmetic dentist, or involve a periodontist or plastic surgeon the dentist partners with.

GUM LIFT

One type of gum alteration is used when there is a little extra gum tissue or asymmetry in gum heights, which calls for a small diode laser that can remove a little extra tissue and tooth here and there until all the gum lines match up. Many veneer cases call for some sort of gum lift to help blend the veneers, as almost everyone has some unevenness in their gum lines, and most cosmetic dentists are trained to do this.

However, sometimes contouring is more complicated. A gum lift may be paired with a crown lengthening procedure, where excess bone along the gum line is removed along with the excess gum. A periodontist would do this more complex pre-procedure.

GUM GRAFT

If the person is experiencing some gum recession—where the gum has fallen back and too much of the tooth root is exposed, perhaps causing sensitivity and the teeth to look really long—we also call in a periodontist to graft and regrow gum tissue to a healthier height. The small bit of tissue needed can be taken from the roof of the patient's mouth, which heals quickly. In other cases, donor tissue is used instead.

LIP REPOSITIONING

Sometimes a person's lips jump up too high, almost to their nose, when they smile. In these cases, we might try Botox injections to relax the lip and keep it from jumping up so high. In a more extreme case, we might make a referral to a facial plastic surgeon who can permanently alter how the lip positions itself.

The combination of procedures you and your dentist decide to use for your smile makeover—including soft tissue adjustments—will, of course, always depend on what's right for you.

GET THE RIGHT SMILE MAKEOVER FOR YOU

There are a lot of options and levels of involvement for any smile makeover. There is no one size fits all; there's just the size that fits you. And you get what you pay for. That's as true in cosmetic dentistry as it is in any other field where medical skills and craftsmanship are important. The *who* of a makeover matters just as much as *what* you end up doing. Take the time necessary to find a dentist you feel confident will work with you the way you want, address your concerns, and who has the skills necessary to create a design and treatment plan that prioritizes *you* and the needs of your smile.

Getting a lot of opportunities to fine-tune your smile before anything permanent is done addresses many of those needs. This means making sure a smile test drive is part of the process a dentist offers.

Bear in mind there's no way to test drive minor makeovers or smile upgrades because they are done quickly and don't involve substantial changes to the teeth—since upgrades are progressive, we check as we go and stop when we all agree the smile is good.

For more major makeovers, though, you'll want that test drive before any big changes take place. And so you know what to look for and expect during this step of the smile makeover process, we're diving into the particulars of the smile test drive next.

94 · CREATING A CONFIDENT SMILE

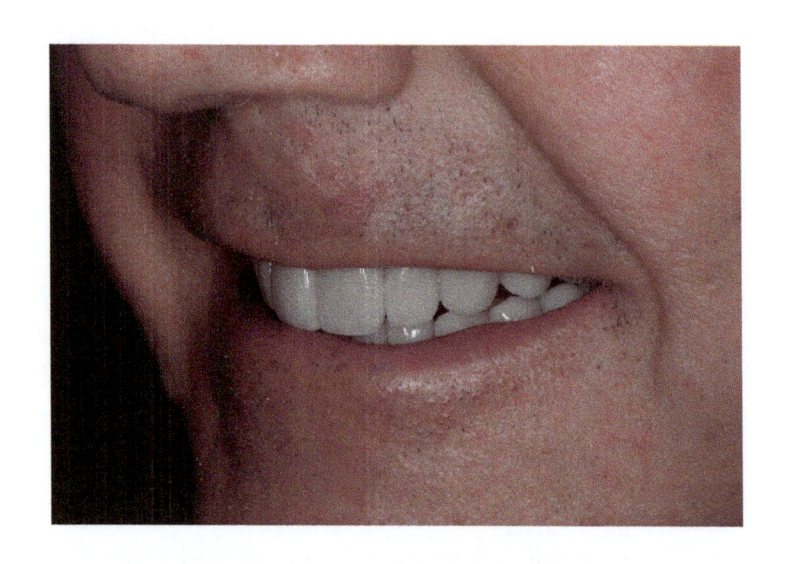

Chapter 5

The Smile Test Drive

"I've always had a lot of issues with my teeth growing up," Hannah told us at her consultation. "Root canal at a very young age, countless cavities, tons of inlays and crowns. The sensitivity just keeps getting worse."

A lot may have happened to her mouth, but the wear on her teeth didn't quite match her actual years. Hannah was a young patient for us. This meant her smile would need to last her a long time. So, we wanted to be especially conservative in her smile design.

Hannah thought she wanted traditional veneers, because she feared her smile might look too bulky with prepless, but we started our test drive appointment with a model of the simpler prepless veneers, just so she could see what they were like.

After seeing and feeling the model of the prepless smile design in her own mouth, Hannah realized they looked nice, indeed, and decided to go with that smile option.

A key to success in the smile design process is being able to test drive your new smile in your mouth before anything becomes permanent. There are many options for a test drive, some of which are related to the type of procedure you receive, but all of them offer the advantage of knowing what your new smile will look and feel like in real life.

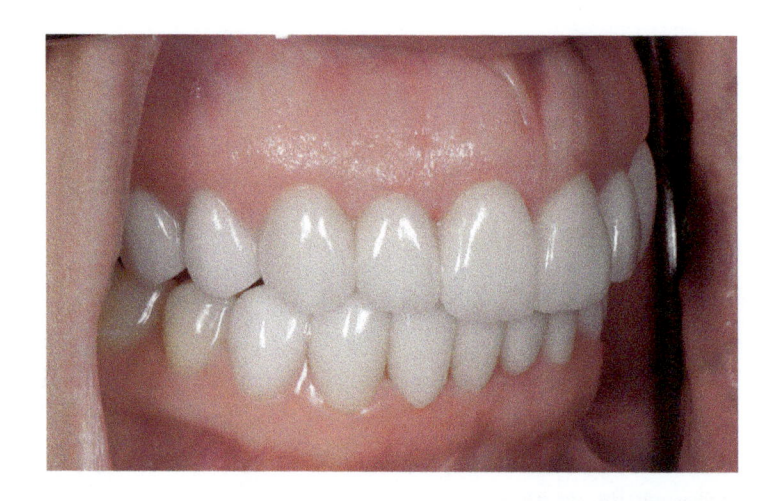

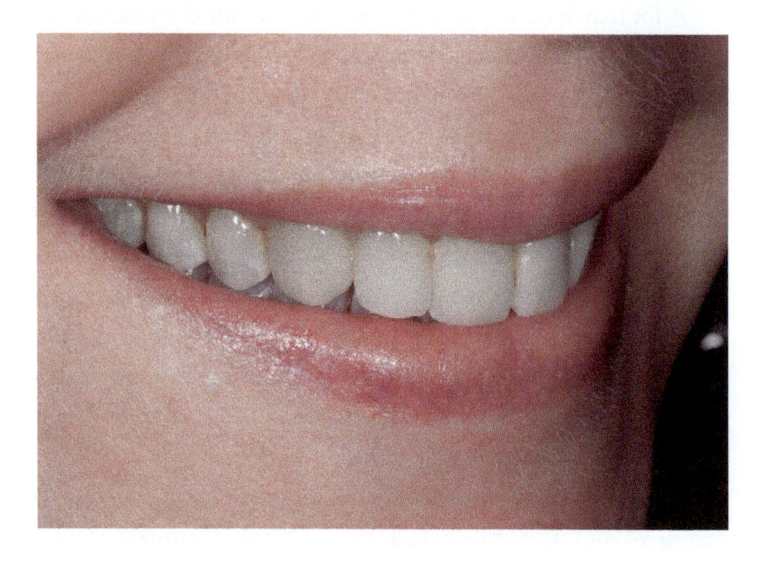

TYPES OF TEST DRIVES: FROM DIGITAL TO ANALOG

The first test drive is digital, and is done in the office in one appointment, after the initial consultation appointment. We use both a digital ideal model of the new smile and a very temporary mock up model you can wear around the office. A combination of scans, photos, and videos digitize your face and mouth, and we import these into our computer-aided design (CAD) software. We use the software to look at your facial features, lip positioning, and movement of the lips and cheeks as you talk. Similar to what an architect might do, we design a digital ideal smile based on your individual features and movements—we work with the space and features of your personal landscape. The ideal model is our blueprint during the design process and represents the new smile.

The digital ideal smile is still an abstract concept, since it's a virtual rendering of your smile and you don't yet have the sensory feedback of physically having that smile in your mouth. Some patients don't resonate much with this mostly hands-off part of the test drive. For others, like those who need a full mouth reconstruction, the CAD design can show more of the reasoning behind each process decision—see under the cheek, so to speak, of what will be done to help their tooth health and bite dynamics. At a minimum, we typically go through a presentation of the whole design process with patients who would benefit from test drives, so they understand each step involved and why it's necessary.

Once the digital ideal smile is designed and approved by the patient, we send it to our computer-aided manufacturing program, the CAM part of CAD/CAM, which prints a physical 3D model. We call this model smile a mock-up. It's made of a malleable resin material that we form in the mouth over the teeth to simulate what the new smile, such as veneers, is going to look like. Since the mock-up is added over the top of the teeth, it's a bit bulkier than the real smile would be. As we'll see in Chapter 8, we do prep work on the teeth at a different point in the process, which makes room for the new porcelain veneers to bond seamlessly to the existing tooth structure. However, the bulkiness of the mock-up lets us see and point out where and how much tooth reduction will be needed to make the new smile comfortable. Once we're done taking more pictures and using the mock up to evaluate and refine the smile, the resin is removed easily, and the patient goes home. Since the resin isn't glued or bonded to the teeth in any way, it only has about an hour of usefulness. The mock-up acts as a rough draft we can edit, and helps us solidify the game plan.

The malleable mock-up model allows us to try out the proposed smile and better understand what needs to be done to complete the smile makeover before we ever touch your actual teeth. It also gives us feedback on what should change.

The first test drive appointment with the digital design and physical mock-up models is a prelude to the third type of test drive we do: the temporary smile. For veneers, as for other makeovers, this happens at the prep appointment, when we do the permanent prep work on the teeth and fabricate plastic temporary veneers out of the same resin material we used for the mock up and then glue them on. The temporary veneers allow you to test drive a newer iteration of your smile more thoroughly. You can see how colors, shapes, lengths of teeth—all the aesthetic options available to you—will look in your actual mouth on a temporary basis. This analog test drive will stay in your mouth for one to four weeks, depending on the case, so you can get used to it. In a follow-up appointment that occurs anywhere from one to seven days later, we check in on how you're doing with the temporaries and use your feedback to make any final tweaks to the smile design for the permanents.

And now a few caveats to the test drive process. Especially

for additive mock-ups, sometimes the teeth are out of place and the visual isn't perfect. That's why also doing the temporary test drive down the line after some initial work has been done, like straightening and prepping, is important to get even closer to what the actual permanent smile will look like.

If you are doing a simpler smile upgrade like straightening, you won't need the second or third type of test drive—the mock-up or the glued-in temporary smile—since we don't remove any tooth material in that procedure. Here, you might only see a digital CAD design. As a reminder, for procedures like whitening, which are progressive over multiple sessions and reverse themselves over time, you won't even need digital designs, as we can check the color as we go.

The mock-up model and temporary smile are relevant for major smile makeover procedures, as outlined in Chapter 4. Again, like all parts of a good smile makeover, the test drive is customizable.

WHY DO A SMILE TEST DRIVE?

Most people like to kick the tires on a new car before they buy it. Your new smile should get no less attention than a car because that car won't be parked in your mouth. Accounting for the fact that a new smile can cost just as much as a car, it's vital to ensure all parties involved are making the right choices in terms of looks, function, and lifestyle. In our humble opinion, test-driving a smile in order to edit the design according to your feedback (it is *your* smile, after all) is a no-brainer.

Despite the benefits they offer to both the dentist and the patient, test drive appointments aren't the norm in many practices. There are a few reasons for this. First, not every dental practice has access to digital design technology, such as CAD/CAM software. Or, they don't have the ability to do 3D printing for the mock-up models.

Second, the appointment adds more time for the dentist, which isn't necessarily factored into the overall price of the smile makeover. It's hard to justify charging people for a test drive, after all, since it's technically still part of the shopping-around process and there's no firm commitment on the part of the patient to move forward with the makeover. A lot of dental practices aren't comfortable with that uncertainty to their bottom line.

The third reason is more simple: the clinician doesn't have the training or technical expertise to do test drives.

So with all of these reasons *not* to do a test drive appointment, why do we do them?

We think anyone who is considering going down the prepless route needs to experience the additional volume in their mouth. "I didn't realize how much bulkier prepless would come out to be," Hannah admitted after hers were done, "but Dr. Field reassured me we could shave down the thickness, which we did, and now I feel more confident with my new teeth!"

Sometimes, patients like the idea of doing a procedure that doesn't take away any of their existing tooth structure, but they change their minds when they actually see and feel what that means for their mouth in action. They realize they don't like bigger or bulkier teeth, and we're able to change directions midway through and go with a smile makeover option that doesn't change their smile's material volume.

For people who are looking at traditional veneers, we can use the test drives to visualize shapes and contours and color *in the person's mouth*. It's the difference between looking at a paint color in the hardware store and seeing it on your living room wall. We want to see how all those design features will look in action, catching the light as you talk and interacting with your active face. The test drive lets us know if we're going in the right direction with the design, or if we need to adjust.

Simply put, we want to get the best results for each individual patient. We want to limit hiccups down the line, when things start getting real. We want our patients to be happy with their smile at the end of the day—not going to another clinic for a fix. We've done our fair share of fixes when the first dentist doesn't deliver and it's never pleasant.

The smile test drive is an investment in the smile design process with our patients. It follows the old adage, "Treat others how you would want to be treated." If we, as dentists, chose to go through a smile makeover ourselves (and some of us have), we would want to have as much knowledge and information as possible going in. We'd also like reassurance that the dentist we're working with is there to act as a collaborator and is willing to listen to us.

Giving you the ability to experience your smile in your mouth takes the guesswork out of smile design. It also takes a lot of the anxiety out of the process as it moves into more intense stages, when we're altering your teeth forever. It's powerful, and empowering, to understand fully, with all of your senses, what this new smile will be like as a part of you. And it helps you more firmly and immediately choose the makeover option that will give you the most mental and physical comfort and confidence moving forward. You don't have to convince yourself that this smile is right for you; you *know* it's right. The test drive makes your future smile more real. And having concrete knowledge about what the end result will be helps motivate you through the more uncomfortable parts of the process.

We want to know if the smile we've designed will accomplish what both you and we want it to accomplish: looks, function, health. In some cases, the verdict is a quick "Yes!" and we can quickly progress to the next step. In other cases, it's a, "No, not quite right," and we have to go back to the drawing board. Knowing that ahead of doing permanent work saves so much time and headache on the backend that the test drive appointment proves its worth.

A SMILE IS FOREVER, SO MAKE TIME FOR A TEST DRIVE

Sometimes less can be more, and the goal is to find what's right for you, not the most expensive or involved procedure available. Without doing a test drive, Hannah would have followed her initial instincts and gone with traditional veneers, which would have looked great, but would have required more prep work on the teeth, which would have limited her later options for restorations when the lifespan of her original veneers ran out.

A smile makeover, especially a major makeover, is forever. There's no going back after prepwork on the teeth begins. Due to both its permanence and prevalence, the smile makeover process should start with a test drive for your own peace of mind. You wouldn't remodel your house without looking at and providing input on the architect's plans. Unless you're appearing on an HGTV program, you wouldn't show up on reveal day, hoping it's what you want. Your smile, a permanent part of you, should be no different.

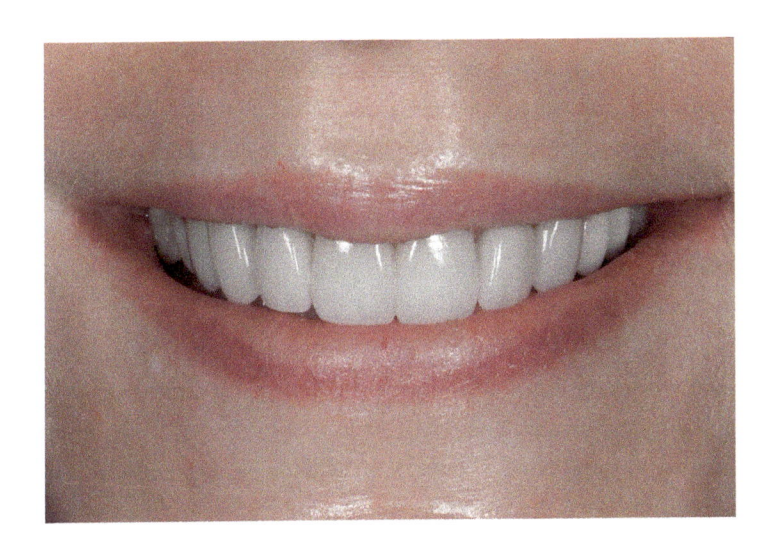

The apparent lack of priority our smiles take compared to other aspects of our lives is a perennial mystery to those of us in the dental field. We suspect the embarrassment or stigma surrounding visibly flawed or damaged smiles makes people feel they have to get their smiles fixed on the sly, like some covert operation—get in, fix it, and get out, hopefully without making eye contact with anyone in the process. But this rush and evasion of the process limits a patient's ability to be *part* of the process, and that lack of ownership can translate to disappointment with their new smile.

A picture's worth a thousand words, but getting the full sensory experience of a test drive is worth more. To feel and try out your new smile in your mouth will give you a personal connection to the treatment plan and just what goes into delivering on that plan. You don't have to put all your faith in what the dentist says it will look like.

The smile test drive involves you playing a role in the creation of your own smile and forges an emotional connection between you and your smile-to-be. It allows you to feel and see what that smile will look like in your own mouth. Pictures taken throughout the process, test drives, and various check-ins assure you that the smile you're being paired with is a lifematch.

Remember, not all dental practices offer test drives, so if this part of the process is important to you, make test drives a part of your criteria when you vet dentists.

Now that you know the type of smile makeover you want and you've tried out and refined the design, it's time to choose the physical materials that will go into creating this smile. Each has its pros and cons, and the type of makeover you choose will determine what type of materials you might need or want.

Chapter 6

Material Options and Impacts

Wendy needed her veneers fixed. A little prophetically, she'd been given a referral to our practice from her orthodontist, but had lost the information. So instead, she went to another dentist who used a more traditional approach to veneers. They took an impression of her teeth and had a lab design the veneers in wax around a stone model.

Many adults are familiar with this approach, and have perhaps even experienced some version of it. But the approach isn't ideal for designing the look of someone's smile. To make it worse, not only were Wendy's veneers created using a copy of her teeth and without the reference point of her real mouth and face, but she also didn't have a lot of involvement in her smile design process. She wasn't given an opportunity to provide feedback about the shape, color, and material of her veneers before the permanents went in. The material choice and execution were especially glaring. The way her ceramic veneers had been made and processed left her new smile looking fake, with no real life to it—characteristics that didn't fit Wendy at all. By this point, knowing how important appearance can be to a smile, it isn't surprising that Wendy ended up in our office for a do-over.

For her smile makeover 2.0, we discussed what her design process would look like, showed her the test drives, and—most importantly for her—went over the material options and application techniques available to her so she could pick the ones that would give her the effect she was going for. This time, we used layered materials that added more sparkle, and she ended up with what she had wanted all along: the smile from her youth.

It's not like Wendy's first dentist did anything wrong. The veneers were functional, applied properly, and looked okay. But traditional cosmetic techniques and materials can't provide the level of design a patient like Wendy needs. Her teeth had broken down a fair amount by the time she got her makeover, and she wanted her veneers to restore the smile she'd had in the past. But her first set of veneers just took their cue from Wendy's current teeth, both in terms of shape and color. In her case, the monolithic, traditional material used to make her first veneers wasn't going to create the look she wanted. She needed a layered mix of materials that would better refract light and de-age her teeth.

Not all materials are created equal. From the brightest pearly whites to the most natural of grins, everyone has different goals for how they want their smile to look and function. The dental material you choose for your makeover carries ramifications for the long-term use and final aesthetics of your smile.

The search for the best material for smile makeovers is never-ending. It's a quest to find materials that can mimic the complex and fascinating properties of real teeth. Teeth are the only substance of the body made to appear on the outside, exposed to the environment and human view, and as such, they combine unique properties of strength, durability, and aesthetics. Again, it's that cross-purpose of health, function, and appearance—natural healthy teeth have it all, so anything we repair them with has to have the same properties and achieve the same outcomes.

Thirty years ago, in the dark days of modern dentistry, none of these properties were available to us. Restorative materials weren't that strong, durable, or pleasing to look at. For example, in the history of our twenty-five-year-old practice, the first materials we commonly used were polymers, a type of plastic. They looked okay, but had a tendency to chip and didn't last very long.

We moved to ceramic materials when technology made it available. These were initially pressed out of monolithic materials—in other words, they were made of one type of substance. They gave us strength and durability and were much better in appearance than plastics. Then we learned how to mill and layer different types of ceramics to make them look so close to real teeth you'd hardly know the difference.

The dental ceramics world is constantly evolving. These materials are highly studied, and new recommendations and techniques are always being added to our repertoire of options. Along with all of our other hats, dentists are manufacturers, so we're always looking for ways to improve ceramics to make them stronger, longer-lasting, and more beautiful. For that reason, we anticipate this chapter will need an update ten, or even five, years from now. Having our own lab means we can get pretty nerdy about the physical materials used to create a permanent smile, but we promise to keep the technical stuff to a minimum.

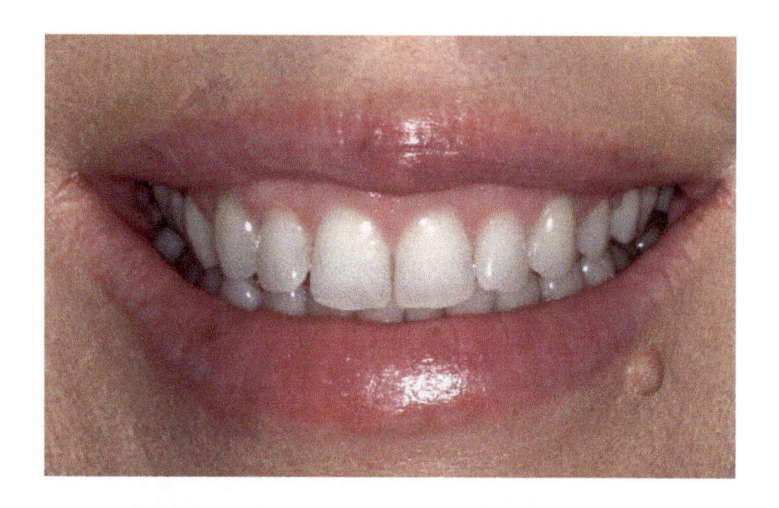

VENEER MATERIALS

Veneers have been around for a few decades at this point, and while there are specific cases that call for the older material of composite plastics, modern veneers usually reside in the world of zirconium or true ceramics. Let's break it down.

CERAMICS

Currently, ceramics are the best materials available and make up the vast majority of veneers. Any material called ceramic consists of a ratio of a powder silicate and a liquid. The main component of ceramics is fine sand—that's the silicate—a natural material that's a cousin to the ceramics used for kitchen sinks and fine china. Like their mundane relatives, dental ceramics, otherwise known as porcelains, go through physical changes when they are worked and fired, becoming hard, strong, and shiny. And best of all, they come in all shades of white—sometimes at the same time if we're using layering, which produces a polychromatic effect.

Think of the translucent, liquid look of white bone china, which contains some of the same types of ceramics as veneers and can show gradations in color depending on the lighting.

The nature of this pure, natural material also means it physically bonds to the prepped tooth structure, molecularly joining with the tooth for a smooth, strong pairing, similar to how porcelain joins to the base metal of sinks or bathtubs. Like these high-end fixtures, the texture of porcelain veneers also has that pearl-smooth, almost liquid quality, which is as close as we can get to the texture of real teeth. This property, as well as the fact that they are natural materials, makes ceramics a very friendly partner to the biological materials of the body. In other words, the body doesn't produce a negative immune reaction to ceramics.

Within ceramics, the two main types used for dentistry are feldspathic porcelain and lithium disilicate, both of which have subtle differences in the properties we want, but overall deliver top-level results.

Feldspathic Porcelain

Out of all the ceramics, feldspathic ceramics have been around the longest—more than twenty years. The optical effects and light properties it produces are the closest to natural teeth, so when we talk about the "prettiest" veneers, feldspathic porcelain is still the winner. Because of the layering technique used to apply it, which builds color gradually, it's easier to match the veneer colors to the existing tooth color. In other words, if a smile design only calls for four veneers in the front, we can blend those veneers into the existing smile so it's difficult to tell which teeth were worked on and which weren't.

The downside of feldspathic ceramics is that they are finicky, and require a highly-skilled and highly-artistic process to create a quality porcelain. Everything—from the smile design, to the layering of the permanent veneers in the lab, to the seating process on the teeth—has to be perfect. They are also relatively fragile compared with other types of veneer materials. Therefore, feldspathic porcelain is only indicated for patients with little to no wear on their old teeth and who don't have any major parafunctional issues, such as clenching or grinding, which put more stress and friction on the veneers.

Lithium Disilicate

If we need something stronger than feldspathic to get the durability and strength we want, we would go with the next step up for ceramic materials: lithium disilicate. This material, mostly used under the trade name of EMAX, accounts for about 70 percent of the veneers done today. It's approximately three times as strong as feldspathic ceramic and holds up to harder use. It's also a little more forgiving on the clinical side, both in terms of fabrication and installation, which means it's easier for the lab partner and dentist to work with, adjust on the fly, and achieve a nice final look.

We say "nice" because, when it comes to cons for lithium disilicate, it just doesn't look as good as feldspathic porcelain. And the technician still has to have a fair amount of skill to layer lithium disilicate—literally painting one thin layer of material after another on top of each other—in such a way as to maximize its aesthetic properties and get it close to the look of feldspathic porcelain.

While using a layering technique isn't essential to get a strong smile, it is important to get one that looks and acts like natural teeth. Teeth, like pearls, are built using thin layers of biological material, a technique that helps give them strength, flexibility, and pearlescence. To produce an accurate mimic of these natural wonders, we ideally need to use the same construction methods as nature. The patient's part in achieving this look means engagement with the process: completing all the appointments for design and test drives, the delivery appointment of the permanent porcelain veneers, and care of the smile afterward. If we need a quicker, cheaper, or less involved option, we can go to composites.

COMPOSITES

Composite materials are polymers, also known as plastics. They are made from a combination of materials that come in a soft state that can be molded and cured easily in the mouth.

Composite materials are what veneers used to be made from, before we had the capability to use ceramics. Because they are not as good as ceramics, they are now more often used as filler material for cavities. Most of us have probably had a dental experience that includes the dental "ray gun" that shoots blue UV light on a tooth the dentist is working on. That's what hardens the polymer.

Overall, polymers are easy and quick to work with. They can be applied in one chair-side visit and are easy to adjust. They are also less expensive than ceramics. But they lack the durability of porcelains, are more prone to chips, stains, and wear, and are not as pretty to look at. Tone-wise, their whiteness can still match the other teeth in the smile, but plastics don't refract light the way ceramics do.

On the opposite end of the spectrum is zirconium, the heavyweight of modern dental materials.

ZIRCONIUM

Zirconium is the strongest of the tooth-colored restorative materials. As a substance, it lives between ceramics and metal, and there's still a lively debate among experts about what side of the periodic table it's closest to. This is because its construction and properties are sometimes similar to ceramics and, at others, similar to metals. For instance, zirconium is about three to four times stronger than lithium disilicate, which is the strongest true ceramic we have. This makes zirconium the absolute best material if you're looking for strength and durability.

However, zirconium trades off its looks for its strength. It has the worst optical properties of any of the veneer materials. It also doesn't bond to teeth the way ceramics do. Like a metal, it needs to be cemented into place, which means smile designs are more aggressive to ensure the zirconium stays fastened to the tooth, extending the prep deeper into the tooth surface and around the sides of the tooth so the zirconium can get a better grip.

When we move to smile designs that require more intense reconstructions, we still use combinations of the same materials, but their durability and strength become even more important.

IMPLANT MATERIALS

While veneers make up the majority of smile makeovers, we also do a fair amount of implants when we have little or no healthy tooth left to work with. When talking about implant materials, we need to look at each part of the implant to determine what's best: the screw, the abutment, or the new tooth.

TITANIUM VS. ZIRCONIUM SCREWS

The screw is the part of the implant that is embedded into the bone of the upper or lower jaw. It acts to replace the missing tooth root and holds the new tooth in place. Unlike dentures, which just float above the gum line, an implant restores bite force and some neural feedback as you eat. You can feel pressure when you bite down with it. When talking about the screws of an implant, the two materials used are titanium and zirconium, both of which are in the metal family. The screw implantation is usually done by an oral surgeon, though some dentists are trained in this procedure. If you have preferences for implant materials, include this specialist as part of your smile makeover discussions.

Titanium is the typical or traditional material used for surgical implants. It's been used in medicine for a long time for other types of physical reconstructions, like hip replacements and the screws that hold metal plates onto fractured bones. One of the main reasons for this is that titanium is inert, meaning it doesn't react to biological material and is very friendly to being used in the body. This long track record of success in medicine makes it a predictable and relatively safe material to use.

However, titanium, as a true metal, is gray. This means that the darker screw may show through at the gum line for people who have thinner gum tissue. And for the few people with full-on metal allergies, titanium can still be uncomfortably reactive and cause an immune response, sometimes being rejected by the body after implantation.

We want to reassure you that this level of metal sensitivity is extremely rare, and the people who have it know long before they walk through our doors that metal is a problem for them, as every piece of metal their skin comes into contact with causes discoloration and dermal flare-ups. But if someone isn't sure, or has had mixed reactions to different metals, there are simple blood or contact tests we can do to make sure the titanium won't be an issue. If we can't use titanium because of these reasons, there is another option.

Zirconium used for implant screws is very similar to the material used for zirconium veneers. Theoretically, it's even more inert than titanium, which is why we use it for metal-sensitive patients. Zirconium, being that hybrid between metal and ceramic, also has the advantage of being tooth-colored. We can fashion the whole implant—screw and tooth—out of it, which means no dark metal shows through the gums.

The one disadvantage of zirconium is that, despite its strength, it isn't quite as strong as titanium, so it does have a higher risk of fracture if put under too much stress. This durability issue makes it a second choice to titanium, mainly only employed in those cases where sensitivity and discoloration are of concern. Another drawback is that it isn't commonly used in mainstream dentistry, so not all dentists are trained and comfortable working with it. If you have a metal sensitivity or are concerned about thinner gums, you'll want to talk to your dentist and oral surgeon ahead of time to see if zirconium is something they use.

TITANIUM VS. ZIRCONIUM ABUTMENTS AND CROWNS

Once the screw is in and the jaw has gone through a healing process, it's time to put in the permanent abutment and crown. Together, these make up the new tooth.

Abutments are the piece of the implant that connects to the screw on one side, and the new tooth on the other. Once you have attached an abutment to an implant screw, the whole structure looks and acts like a tooth that's been prepared for a crown—in short, you have a small metal tooth sticking out of your gum. The last part of the implant, the crown or visible tooth, clicks and cements onto the abutment and extends from the gum line to the biting edge of the tooth. The crown will look like a normal tooth.

Abutments can also be made out of titanium or zirconium, with the same properties as for the screws applying here. This is where the coloration problem of titanium can come into play, as the abutment interfaces with the gum in the visible zone between the jaw bone and new tooth, so we are very selective when we use titanium for this part of the implant. For example, if we are replacing a back molar for a person who has a heavy bite and lots of clenching or grinding, we'll go with the stronger titanium. Otherwise, if we're working on the front of the mouth, we want to use zirconium.

This leads us right to the last type of makeover and list of materials: those used for the crowns.

CROWN MATERIALS

Crowns are one of the oldest types of smile makeovers, and as such, a rich and diverse array of materials have been used to construct them over time. The materials we will discuss in this section are currently used for both implant crowns that seat over the implant screws and regular crowns that seat over prepared existing teeth. We'll go through these materials historically, starting with the most ancient materials used for crowns and ending with the most modern.

GOLD

We know those of you who've seen *Home Alone*—where one of the Wet Bandits loses his favorite gold tooth to Kevin's defensive paint cans—might be wondering, where's my gold tooth? To satisfy any lingering curiosity, here are the origins of this old favorite.

Gold's been a mainstay of ornamentation in the archeological record for as long as civilization has existed. It's shown up in dentistry for at least as long as history records dental practices. There's evidence the ancient Egyptians used it thousands of years ago in crowns—as in, the ones that go in your mouth—to help reinforce teeth. And it's not surprising they'd use gold for this purpose, because its properties are obvious: it's very biologically friendly, it's infinitely malleable and easy to work with on tiny levels, and it effectively supports and protects teeth.

Gold is rarely used in dentistry anymore for two reasons. One, we have better materials. Pure gold is too soft to hold up in the mouth, so it's always combined in an alloy with some other metal, like nickel, to harden it and give it durability. These other metals are more reactive to body tissue, and can make some people uncomfortable. If you have skin reactions to gold jewelry, it's not the gold that's at fault, but the nickel.

Two, there's little demand for the shiny showpieces that earn famous hip-hop artists and pirates so much fascinated attention. Most want their new teeth to look like teeth. In all our years of cosmetic practice, we've done exactly one gold grill. Embedding diamonds in ceramic veneers is only slightly more common.

We mention gold here mainly because it has such a long history in dentistry, but delving into the world of precious metals and gems and rarer higher-end evolutions of materials takes us out of the types of smile makeovers the majority of our patients want. We also want to mention gold because there are those unique individuals who like the aesthetic properties of gold and want it featured in their smile. As good cosmetic dentists, it's our job to provide our patients with all the pros and cons of the material, show them what it will look like, and then make their dream smile look like a million bucks, with or without the diamonds.

SILVER

We're going to do a quick note on silver, because some of you may remember or still sport old silver fillings. Silver isn't used in modern dentistry anymore because, (1) dental silver has mercury in it to make it malleable, and we know now mercury isn't good for human bodies, and (2) we have better materials. If silver comes up at all in a dentist's office, it's to remove and replace it. There are some materials still in use that look like silver, such as stainless steel for caps and crowns, but these are almost exclusively used in pediatric dentistry, where a quick fix will keep a child's baby tooth functional until it's replaced by a healthy adult tooth.

PFM (PORCELAIN FUSED TO METAL)

From gold, dentistry progressed to PFM, or porcelain fused to metal. We wanted to make the new teeth look more like real teeth but still wanted the strength of the gold, so the inner part of the crown is made from a gold alloy, and then a ceramic is stacked or baked onto the metal to create the shape and color of a real tooth. The advantage here, of course, is a tooth-colored tooth. The disadvantage is that the fuse point between metal and ceramic creates a weak link in the crown structure that can cause chips or breakage as the crown ages. Fortunately, if the porcelain part of the crown pops off, the metal underneath stays attached so that no part of the old tooth abutment is exposed, but it's not an ideal situation to have to go back to your dentist to reattach or make a new crown just because you bit into an apple.

PFMs have been used consistently and routinely for well over thirty years, and there are a lot of practices that still use them as standard care because that's what they were trained to do. Mostly, we see these on the back teeth, because the dark lines along the gums created by the metal showing through the porcelain don't look that great. But sometimes dentists will choose function over aesthetics and put this material on the front teeth, as well.

CERAMICS

As with veneers, ceramics are also commonly used for crowns in modern cosmetic dentistry, especially when the aesthetic property is important, like with front teeth. We don't normally use feldspathic porcelains because crowns need to be stronger than veneers, since they replace the entire outside portion of the tooth. However, we do use lithium disilicate on a regular basis. As a recent advantage, we can now use CAD/CAM technology to make crowns for back teeth in-office during a single appointment, which gives us the ability to deliver a higher quality crown in a reasonable amount of time.

ZIRCONIUM

The part metal, part ceramic nature of zirconium makes it an excellent choice for crowns. As a monolithic material, there's no layering or fusing involved—the crown is one solid piece—so you don't have the weak link problem. Its metal-like properties give it a similar strength to gold, while its ceramic-like properties make it more aesthetically pleasing. Again, zirconium isn't *as* pretty as true ceramics, but it's great for molars and teeth that aren't as visible.

The smile makeover you chose dictates which materials will create your smile. As in any other stage of the smile makeover process, there are a few general things to consider when choosing what your new smile will be made out of. Be aware that all the materials we discussed previously (except for silver) are safe and effective options to use in dentistry, and all will restore health to the mouth. The rest of the selection process depends upon which material properties you and your dentist prioritize in conjunction with your unique smile needs.

GENERAL CONSIDERATIONS WHEN CHOOSING MATERIALS

When we talk about the look of the smile, we're talking about the optical properties of materials, instead of the mechanical properties that pertain to durability and longevity. While optical properties often preoccupy our patients, as dentists, we do want to make sure the new smile lasts a long time.

For dentists, longevity and durability often come first in the conversation about which materials to use in a specific makeover. The reason we start with these properties is because, practically speaking, smile makeovers can be expensive. Many patients want a smile that will last for a long time without needing repairs. These priorities then guide dentists toward stronger materials or techniques, like using a monolithic material such as zirconium, which can make up the entire reconstructed tooth. Then, we might have a patient who wants a balance between durability and looks, which leads us toward lithium disilicate. If looks are a bigger priority and durability isn't necessary for function, then that means feldspathic porcelain.

For some people, keeping as much of their natural teeth as possible is important to them. If a patient has healthy teeth overall but just wants a cosmetic upgrade, we wouldn't recommend full crowns or zirconium veneers; instead, we'd want to do a ceramic veneer that would provide the same longevity when paired with healthy oral habits. Since ceramics and polymers are bonded onto the teeth, we can be more conservative in tooth preparation, sometimes without needing to remove any of the original tooth at all.

Health can also be a factor when we're weighing durability against conserving tooth structure. It follows that someone who needs the durability of a material like zirconium because of a grinding issue probably doesn't have to worry too much about existing tooth structure being removed, because constant grinding has already created a situation where there's not much left to preserve.

Finally, if cost is an issue in the selection process, it may be obvious that the stronger, prettier materials that require specialized training are going to be more expensive. Polymers and monolithic materials cost a little less because they don't require the additional design, skill, and finesse that layered materials do.

At our practice, the policy is to charge the same no matter what material is being used, but this isn't universal among dentists. It's easier for us to maintain this policy because we have our own lab in-house, but most dentists work with an outside lab and ceramist, and rates may differ. To us, it's important that cost doesn't drive your clinical decisions—you shouldn't have to sacrifice the quality of your healthcare and your peace of mind over budget—and material choice should come down to the best material based on your unique case.

You don't want your smile to break down on you. If you go through all the effort and expense to improve it, you want your smile to keep pace with your life. A good dentist will walk you through the process of choosing material types so you can look good, feel good, and have your new smile last a long time.

We've evolved our knowledge to the point where dental materials can do pretty close to what natural teeth do. Still, ceramics need to be handled properly and skillfully by both the lab technician who makes them and the dentist who applies them to achieve the maximum success they offer. It's always a good idea to ask to see photos of restorations done with the materials offered to you and to ask questions about how they will perform and look in your mouth. And, of course, you'll want to know about the process the practice will use to achieve your permanent smile.

Now that we have the smile makeover chosen, planned, and its materials picked, it's time to get into the appointments that will deliver your new permanent smile. First, we'll ease some of the inevitable fears that come with climbing into the dental chair by explaining how we can make the process more comfortable.

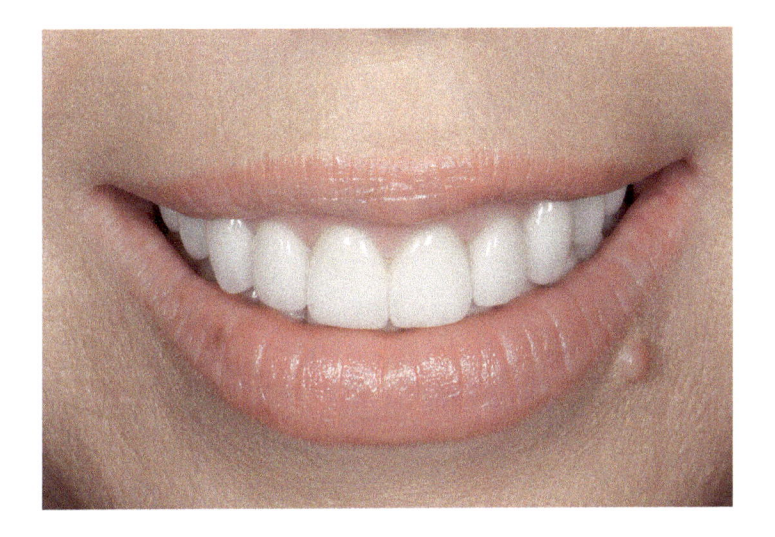

Chapter 7

Making You More Comfortable in the Dental Chair

The majority of this book may be written from a team perspective, taking all the practice's collective knowledge into account, but this next story is mostly mine.

As children, my younger brother and I made hand-to-hand combat a frequent pastime in our home. One of those events got a little out of hand. Let's just say, I had to make a hasty retreat from the battlefield with two chipped lower front teeth.

Over the years, the chips were repaired numerous times with a bonding technique that only had a lifespan of three to five years. Eventually, I got tired of needing to go to the dentist to fix it. I knuckled down and did what many of our patients do: I took some time to invest in my own teeth. I figured I was a cosmetic dentist, after all, and had no excuse not to; plus, I looked a little silly by putting off the work. So, I had one of my partner dentists put in porcelain veneers on my lower front teeth.

While the design process and test drives went fine, I was nervous going into the big prep and permanent appointments. I knew the process by heart and, like many doctors, I have control issues surrounding my own specialty, which can make me a horrible patient. For as much as I love being beside the dental chair, I hate being in it.

To ease my tension, we decided I needed a little help from some mild sedatives used commonly in dental practice, namely the familiar nitrous oxide and the not-so-familiar oral sedative of Valium. The Valium took the edge off, and though I was aware my partner was working on my mouth, I didn't care enough to micromanage. While these sedatives made my time in the chair tolerable, if my partner had been trained to do IV sedation at the time, I would have done that. Then, I could have comfortably drifted on the edges of sleep and not thought about the procedure at all. I'm certified for that premier kind of sedation, but the dental board doesn't look too kindly on dentists sedating themselves—for obvious reasons.

In the end, I was happy with the result. My veneers are about six years old now, and I've had no issues—and, of course, they look great. But getting them would have been much more difficult both mentally and physically if I hadn't had the option of sedatives to keep me calm and comfortable.

Part of the reason I did extra training on sedation techniques was so that I could help people like me, whose normal levels of anxiety and need for control don't allow for a smooth clinical process. Since smile makeovers also impact appearance, which comes with its own brand of stress, the anxiety experienced by some during cosmetic procedures can be more severe than it is during run-of-the-mill dental work, like having cavities filled. Having been there myself, I'm mindful of the strain and compounding discomfort caused by sitting in one position with your mouth open for up to four hours, as can be the case in more involved reconstructions. I get that the dental chair is not the most fun place to be, and I want to make it a better experience for my patients.

People fear going to the dentist, and this fear can be a big roadblock to getting them in that dental chair. Since veneers are also one of the more involved processes, their delivery can carry more anxiety than quick in-and-out fixes. Luckily, there are many technical options for the delivery of your smile that make the process less stressful and uncomfortable.

To be clear, the goal of using sedation during routine dental procedures is not to keep the patient from "escaping," or to amuse the dentist. The real purpose is to take the edge off any minor pain, discomfort, or anxiety that comes from anticipating and going through a procedure that alters and fixes a socially sensitive and functionally essential part of the body. Especially for the procedures that prep the teeth and deliver the permanent smile, a little pharmaceutical relaxation can make the procedure go more smoothly and quickly, and result in less discomfort afterward.

In general, we want the patient to be aware at the end of the appointment to give us feedback on their smile's look and feel, so we'll titrate the dosage, administering small amounts as we go to maintain the desired sedative effect. This means when we stop the doses, the patient recovers quickly and can talk to us by the end of the appointments. And if a patient doesn't like the idea of any type of pharmaceutical, there are some comfort options that require no drugs at all.

Contrary to popular belief, pain is not the main cause of discomfort in the dental chair. Though we will admit, getting shots in the mouth is not on anyone's bucket list and being sedated before those topical analgesics are given can make someone's day a whole lot better. Instead, what gets to many people is the environmental stimuli, which can increase stress levels over time. Sitting in one spot for hours with your mouth open, hearing the noise of the dental tools, feeling water and dust fly at your face as teeth and materials are prepped and shaped, having a bright light shine in your eyes even through the sunglasses provided, and people hovering all around—the whole thing can be mentally, emotionally, and physically taxing. Some people even carry post-traumatic stress from prior dental experiences in which these stimuli weren't managed properly. Even though good dentists will try to limit these stimuli as much as possible, we can't *not* work on your mouth, and that's when comfort options can assist with muting those stimuli.

Below, we've run through the list of ways we can alleviate discomfort during procedures, as well as provided recommendations to help with any post-procedure discomfort.

SELF-HYPNOSIS AND MEDITATION

Very rarely, a patient will come in who has deep experience in self-hypnosis or relaxing themselves with meditation practices. Or, they just have a high discomfort and pain tolerance and zero fear of dental procedures. Especially for shorter procedures, these types of people may need no outside help to remain relaxed and calm. For patients who insist on no pharmaceutical sedation but aren't zen masters, we can also use other types of distractions, like putting on a movie or audiobook, using a guided meditation app, or giving them noise-canceling headphones.

However, for longer procedures, people typically take us up on the offer of a clinical sedative.

LOCAL ANESTHETICS

The most common agent for making patients more comfortable is local anesthetics, or drugs that inject just under the skin and block nerves to create numbness. Their use is standard procedure and ensures no pain comes from the actual work on the teeth or gums.

Articaine, a cousin of the older dental Novocaine many people are familiar with, is the more evolved numbing agent we use today. Like Novocaine and lidocaine, another analgesic in current usage, it's administered under the gums around the teeth that will be getting prepwork or delivery work done. Articaine has a faster onset, longer duration, and bigger effect than other members of the 'caine family of drugs, so after the shots kick in, you may feel some pressure from the work we do to your teeth and gums, but that should be the only thing you feel. After analgesics, we get into true sedatives, starting with the mildest, nitrous oxide.

NITROUS OXIDE

Nitrous oxide, better known as laughing gas because it can make some people giggle, is a combination of oxygen and nitrogen, two elements commonly found in regular old air. A common misconception from movies is that laughing gas can make you pass out, but in real life the patient taking it is very much awake and able to understand and respond to what the dental team is telling them. You know what's going on around you, but you care a little less. This means we still get the advantage of patient involvement in the process, without the disadvantage of patient stress.

Because it is breathed in through a nosepiece, nitrous oxide takes effect within a minute or two, and the dosage can be adjusted in real time. This also means it leaves the body quickly once the gas is taken away. We typically switch to giving the patient pure oxygen when we wrap up the appointment, flushing out what little nitrous oxide is left. Most people are even able to drive their cars home afterward, and that makes it a good option for people who have procedures done in the morning or middle of the day and have to go back to work afterward.

For people who have sensitivities to anesthetics, nitrous oxide is also the most friendly in terms of side effects. Rarely do people get nauseated or dizzy from it, because it contains a mix of gasses the body is used to breathing anyway, just in a different ratio. It's so safe, in fact, that pediatric dentists can use it to calm young children who are getting fillings.

The downside of nitrous oxide is that it's so mild it has the least effect of any sedation option. For people who are extremely nervous or fearful going into a procedure, it can have zero impact. As experienced clinicians, we can easily spot patients who will need a bit more support than nitrous oxide, which is when we move to other options. It also isn't good for longer procedures that last beyond forty minutes, because its effects decrease over time. In these cases, we'll move to other options if a sedative is indicated.

ORAL SEDATIVES

When we need something a little stronger than nitrous oxide, we'll add an oral sedative into the mix because it tends to play well with the gas. Normally, this sedative will be one of a standard line-up of drugs that make people a little sleepy: Valium, Triazolam, or some type of benzodiazepine. If laughing gas mimics the effect of one glass of wine, these drugs are like three of four glasses.

Oral sedatives can make longer and more complex procedures much easier to sit through. However, they do come with a few downsides. Since the drugs are administered orally, it can take a few hours to work their way out of the body's systems, which leaves the person groggy and impaired after the procedure. Because oral sedatives are stronger than nitrous oxide, we do insist the patient brings a driver to take them home after the appointment so the sedative can wear off.

Also, because it's a pill, we can't control the dosing as finely as we can with gas. We have to give the whole suggested dose and wait as it goes through the body and shows its effects. Because the effects are not instantaneous as it works through the GI tract, if the dose doesn't appear to be enough halfway through the procedure, it may be a moot point to give the patient more, as the procedure might be close to done by the time the additional drug takes effect.

Oral sedatives are not foolproof, and they're not 100 percent effective. There is one more option, however, that does give us the power of oral sedatives but more of the dosing control of gas.

INTRAVENOUS SEDATIVES

Intravenous sedation, IV for short, is all about control. It's done in a very controlled environment, and allows us to measure medications exactly. Because the drugs are administered directly into the bloodstream via an IV port in the arm, we know in real time how a medication is affecting the body and can adjust for higher or lower doses as necessary over a very controlled and steady interval that can be maintained for hours. Plus, at the end of a procedure, we can give medications through the IV that can help prevent infection and minimize swelling and pain. This makes it the preferred option for patients with longer or more intense procedures, like a full set of veneers or implants.

The drugs most commonly used in IVs include the same drugs used in oral sedatives, such as benzodiazepines, but these are usually supplemented with an opiate narcotic. The two types of drugs work synergistically to decrease discomfort, stress, and any pain that might come from the procedure. And as a reassurance, we know opiates have come under intense scrutiny because of their abuse outside clinical settings, but since these are dental procedures and we need the patient aware enough to respond to us, the dosing is not as much as it might be in other surgical settings, and we aren't sending patients home with prescriptions for it, since the pain experienced after a well-executed restorative procedure is minimal. It does take a little while for these types of sedatives to leave the body, so as with oral sedatives, a driver and at-home recovery period is needed.

The one caveat to IVs is that they require a clinician trained in how to use and administer them, training which goes beyond the relatively simple training involved for nitrous oxide or oral sedatives. In many clinics, this means the dentist must work with a licensed anesthesiologist, which can prove a little tougher for scheduling since a third party needs to be involved in the appointment. In some practices, the dentist may elect to go through the advanced training required to get IV certification, which makes things much easier for everyone.

Sedation for medical procedures is a given. People expect it as part of the process. But we don't often think about providing ourselves the same comfort options when we get our teeth worked on, even though those procedures can last for the same amount of time and have the same amount of activity and stress as some surgical appointments. For those dentists who have surgical training, offering sedation for patients is part of their early training, but that norm does not exist across the industry. Even those of us trained in restorative work are not automatically trained in more advanced forms of sedation, and many dentists simply don't think about it or have the opportunity to incorporate it as part of their practice. If more advanced sedation techniques are important to you, ask if those options are available as part of your first consultation.

This wraps up the comfort options available during procedures, which is where the vast amount of potential discomfort would be experienced. But there are a few things we can do and recommend to limit any post-procedure swelling and localized pain, too.

ANTI-INFLAMMATORY DRUGS

Permanent smiles shouldn't cause long-term discomfort. But any time we work on teeth and jiggle the nerves in the roots and gums around, there's bound to be a small inflammatory reaction. Therefore, expect a few days of sensitivity post-procedure. After this initial inflammatory response settles with time and a little ibuprofen, the permanent restorations should feel just like normal teeth when in use. For those with sensitive teeth to begin with, smile makeovers like veneers will even help protect the existing teeth they are bonded to and reduce sensitivity.

It's worth mentioning here that the current dental literature says ibuprofen, found in Advil and Motrin, is the most effective pain reliever for dental pain. This is why, though we use heavier drugs for sedation during procedures, we don't usually prescribe them for home use. Acetaminophens like Tylenol, it turns out, are not the best for dental pain.

However, in procedures where the bone structure of the tooth root is affected, like in true orthodontics where braces are involved and embedding implant screws, acetaminophen becomes the better option. This is because ibuprofen interferes with bone healing, which we do not want to do when we're moving teeth around. So for orthodontic discomfort, we recommend acetaminophen. It's not as effective at reducing the pain, but it's more friendly to the healing process, and the good thing is that orthodontic pain is almost always transient. You feel a spike immediately after an adjustment, but it goes away once the teeth adjust to the new alignment asked of them.

While discomfort after the permanent smile is installed should be limited to just a few days of general soreness and can be alleviated by over-the-counter pain medications, we will warn you that temporary smiles can be more problematic—that's why they are temporary.

Not all smile makeovers have temporary smiles you must live with for a few weeks as part of the design process, but both prepped and prepless veneers almost always get a temporary version to test drive. They are made from plastic and are connected together to give them a bit more strength. This construction does not make them feel very natural in the mouth, as the permanent veneers bonded to individual teeth will, and living with them can be a challenge. Temp plastic also doesn't provide the thermal protection the permanent veneer material will, so the newly prepped teeth might experience more sensitivity to hot or cold foods and beverages. For those who find the temps uncomfortable after a couple of days of adjustment, either acetaminophen or ibuprofen works well.

Temporary veneers are a necessary evil that may need some comfort options to make them palatable. We apply desensitizing agents between the prepped teeth and the temporary veneers during the appointment, which helps, but there may be some additional swelling and minor discomfort after other sedatives used during the appointment wear off.

The important thing to remember when talking about discomfort is that, like those plastic teeth, *it's temporary*. Your permanent smile will not hurt or feel weird at all, and if it does, that's something to bring up in the follow-up appointment. And if you've been experiencing mouth and jaw discomfort because of broken down teeth and other health issues, the minor clinical discomfort will be well worth the total relief of having a healthy bite and smile afterward. You might not even realize how much chronic discomfort and pain you've been dealing with in the background until it goes away.

The fleeting discomfort you feel sitting in the dental chair can be mitigated by a number of options. The process can be made practically pleasant. So don't let the fear of discomfort stop you from getting the smile you want.

And that's where we head next: the appointments that get you your permanent smile. Since veneers are most common, we'll use that as an example to lay out this part of the smile makeover process. But know that other types of smile makeovers will follow a similar path.

Chapter 8

The Veneer Clinical Process

We saw Susan about five years before she got her veneers.

When she first came to see us, she admitted that fixing her smile was something she'd been wanting to do for more than a decade, but her nerves had kept her from moving forward. She'd had multiple traumatic dental experiences in the past, and her anxiety around it was now almost unmanageable for her.

"I was terrified," she said later in a testimonial, "and tired of dentists who dismissed my fears without taking the time to fully understand my mouth, my teeth, my overall health, and more importantly, how one impacted the others."

We tried to allay her fears, but the thought of the amount of work to be done overwhelmed her, and she disappeared from our radar.

Five years later, she came back in, and her old smile was getting worse by the day. She now *had* to do something because of basic health concerns—and her daughter's upcoming wedding. But fear still kept her frozen. "It had gotten to the point where I could not even sit in the dentist's chair without physically shaking," she admitted. "Honestly, it's a wonder I did not loosen the chair from the floor."

We spent a lot of time going through the entire smile makeover process with her to help calm her fears. We shared how sedation options could help support her through the more intense parts. She chose IV sedation for both of her major clinical appointments. When the whole thing was done and her new smile in place of the old, she said, "That was the best dental experience I've ever had. I don't know why I waited so long. I wish I would have done this a decade ago."

Getting a new smile is a process, from being able to climb into the chair to seeing your new smile light up a room.

After you've given the go ahead to your dentist following the digital and mock-up test drives and decided on comfort options, we're ready to get down to business of the actual smile makeover. Porcelain veneers take up the majority of a cosmetic dentist's time, and odds are they are your best design option for a makeover. However, they are probably the makeover you're least familiar with, so the procedures to get them need some explaining.

In this chapter, we'll walk through the process from the point of no return—the prep appointment when we get the teeth ready to receive the permanent veneers—through the temporary veneer test drive, to the delivery and follow-up appointments. By the end of this chapter, any concerns you have with the delivery part of the process should be eased as you learn what to expect in the dental chair.

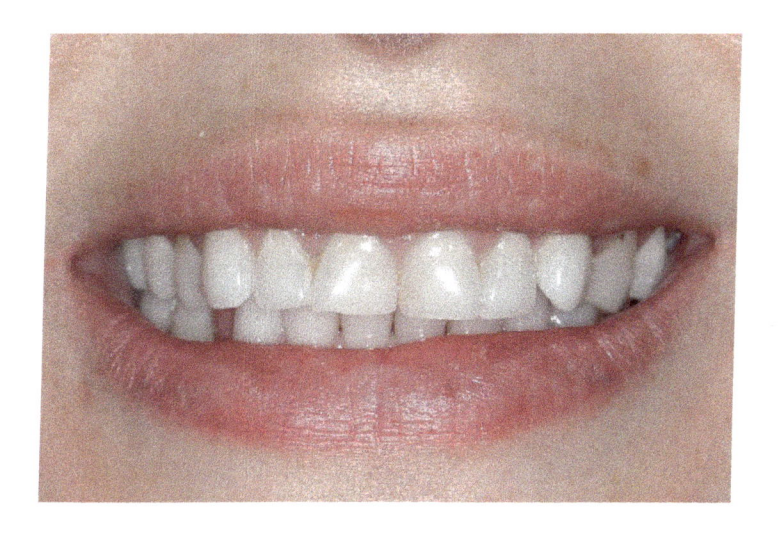

FIRST CLINICAL APPOINTMENT: PREPPING THE SMILE AND TEST DRIVING WITH TEMPORARY VENEERS

The first clinical appointment comes when you sit in the dental chair and get real work done on your teeth and mouth, as opposed to the consultation and test drives that just go over your existing teeth. This is a longer and more involved appointment, anywhere from two to five hours, depending on how many teeth we're doing.

As with the seat appointment we'll discuss next, we recommend consulting with your dentist about comfort options during this first clinical appointment. We encourage you to be proactive here since some dentists are more prone to downplaying this appointment, and sedation and comfort for the patient are not as prominent on their to-do list. Even though there's not a lot of pain associated with the prep appointment, it is still a long time to be sitting in a chair with a team of people scurrying about. If you're interested in one of the comfort options discussed in the previous chapter, this conversation will happen in the initial consultation, because the dentist will need to prepare any necessary medications before the start of the prep appointment.

Now, here's the basic timeline for the appointment itself. Be aware that this timeline follows the steps we see with a majority of our veneer cases, but each case is different, and there may be small changes or exceptions depending on your individual circumstances and procedures.

REVIEW AGENDA

The first thing we'll do when you come in for your prep appointment is sit down and review the plan for the day: what we're going to do to your mouth and teeth and which sedation options we'll be using, if any. This is also a chance for you to ask any questions you might have about the process.

GET YOU COMFORTABLE

After the review, we'll get you seated and comfortable in the dental chair. If you've opted for an oral sedative that needs time to work, you might have already taken one dose at home the night before, and one about an hour before the appointment started. If the comfort plan includes an IV sedation, the port will be put in and a drip started. If you choose nitrous oxide, we'll start those doses with a nosepiece. We'll offer sunglasses and audio options to limit the dental sights and sounds of the room. Once you are suitably relaxed, we'll administer the local anesthetic—articaine or lidocaine—to numb up the area we'll be working on. When that takes effect, we get to work.

GUM CONTOURING

If it's applicable to your smile design, the first bit of work we'll do is gum contouring, otherwise known by dentists as gingival architecture. As we talked about in Chapter 4, this only pertains to minor gum lifts, where we use a fine laser to remove tiny amounts of extra tissue to reshape the gums so they are even across the gum line. More involved procedures like gum grafts, which are done for recession, and crown lengthening, which removes excess bone, are addressed at an earlier appointment with a periodontist and require a small healing period. Note that some dentists may work with a periodontist to do any kind of gum work.

PREP TEETH BY REMOVING DAMAGE, DECAY, AND OLD DENTAL WORK

Once we've dialed in the soft tissue of the gums, we'll do the dental version of a "demo day" by removing all the bad stuff in your mouth. Failing veneers, crowns, or fillings will be removed, and we'll grind away decay and damage until we're back to healthy tooth structure. We'll know from all our early design prep and scans just what to expect here, and we'll follow our conservative approach to only take off as much as we need to in order to restore proper health, function, and appearance with the new smile.

As we're removing the old, we'll also prep the teeth for the new. Depending on which materials we're using for the new veneers, we'll shape the teeth to make the bonding strong and the color seamless with the biological teeth. If other procedures like fillings or crowns are involved in the smile design, we'll prep for and put them in at this point in the process, since those can be done chairside.

CHECK THE WORK

After the gums and teeth are prepped and ready to get their veneers, we'll check our work with a new set of digital scans using our CAD technology to make sure we've done all we need to do. These scans also give us what we call a working model, 3D printed using the CAM computer, upon which we build the new veneers. This process replaces the goopy impression material many people are uncomfortably familiar with when it overflows its trays and causes them to gag.

Once the internal scans for the working model are taken, we take external photographs of the color of the prepped teeth so we can more precisely match the veneer color to the existing tooth color, if that's the look we're going for. For porcelain materials, this matching is where the artistry comes in. Since porcelains have that translucent, pearl-like quality, the natural tooth color will show through to some extent and influence the color of the porcelain. This will determine what kind of mix and layering we do to account for the tooth the porcelain will be paired with so we can get the color and look of the smile we've designed.

In addition to the shape and color of the teeth, we'll also check how our work has impacted your bite, so we'll get another set of bite impressions to update our record and make any tweaks to the shape of the teeth necessary to ensure proper alignment. This is one of the reasons we only want a limited form of sedation; it's easier to get these records when the patient has the awareness to participate and follow requests. We'll stop sedation at a certain point in the appointment so by the time we're ready for you to give us more active feedback on the look and fit of your smile, you'll be awake and aware enough to participate.

MAKE AND ATTACH THE TEMPORARY VENEERS

With updated models and records in hand, we can now make the temporary veneers using a template based on the digital working model. As a reminder, the temporary veneers are made out of the same plastic material used for the earlier mock-up model, only this time they are glued onto the prepared teeth using a temporary cement that will last throughout the test drive process. They'll feel like a clear plastic retainer, if you've ever experienced that piece of orthodontic equipment. Despite their awkwardness and ho-hum looks compared with the final veneers, the temporaries will be more comfortable than the bulky mock-up model worn in the first test drive because we're now replacing and idealizing the volume we've removed from the original teeth. The increased comfort is good, because you'll be wearing them for two to three weeks as we use the temps to evaluate and refine the smile design.

Since the glue isn't as strong and the plastic doesn't bond to the teeth the way the final veneers will, the temps are also constructed with the veneers connected together. This makes them harder to floss and keep clean. We'll advise how to do this at this point in the process. Although the maintenance for temporaries is more involved, it's important to keep the gums and mouth healthy so we don't have any additional health complications during the final install.

The bite will be checked again once the temps are in place, and an impression will be taken in order to make a protective retainer you'll wear with the temporaries when sleeping. Because of their relative fragility, the temps need to be protected from the weird things people often do with their teeth and jaws while dreaming. You'll also need to watch what you eat. No whole apples, chewy breads, or sticky candy that can pop off the temps! We don't want another appointment to reattach or fix the temps just a few days into the test drive.

And though we harp on temporaries a little because some patients find them to be the hardest part of the process, other patients aren't bothered by them at all. If you fall in the former category, know that the evil of temps is necessary because the information they give us helps make the permanent veneers so very good.

TEMPORARY VENEER FOLLOW-UP

Anywhere between one day and a week later, you can expect to come in for a follow-up appointment where we check how the temporaries are responding as they live in your real mouth. It takes a little while for the inflammation and stiffness from the prep appointment to recede, so we want to see how the veneers feel and look in your mouth when everything is at its normal baseline. We'll ask some questions: Are the shapes okay? How is the color blending with your other teeth when in other types of light? Are you experiencing any uncomfortable bite issues when you eat or rest? If you're out of the area, or only have simple feedback or a thumbs-up on fit, the follow-up can be done via a video call, where we can see how the temps look and take some screenshots for reference.

It's important to have this dialogue after the temps have been worn for a while, because you'll have a good idea of what to expect from the permanent veneers. If there's a problem with the function or aesthetics, we want to fix it. We want to make all the modifications we can before your new smile is installed, so you can hit the ground grinning. And it gives you a chance to adjust to the new smile and know what to expect.

Temporaries are just that—temporary. Data we gather at the follow-up will be noted and applied to the final preparation of the permanent veneers, which will take a week or two to make in the lab after the temp follow-up, depending on the number of veneers and the complexity of other restorations needed, such as crowns. Temps are the last and most complete draft we have before the final is due, and so they give us our best chance to make any big changes—to color, to shape, to size—before we're locked into the smile you'll be living with long term.

Which brings us to the main event: the delivery appointment in which your new smile becomes a permanent part of you.

SECOND CLINICAL APPOINTMENT: DELIVERING YOUR NEW CONFIDENT SMILE

Within about two to three weeks total after the temporaries go in, you'll come back to have them removed and the permanent veneers installed.

FINAL REVIEW OF SMILE DESIGN

Much like the first clinical appointment where the prep work is done and temporaries are put in, the second appointment starts with a review. This time, we look at the final veneers, bridge, or implants on "the last working model"—your own mouth—for a last confirmation that this is the smile you want.

GET YOU COMFORTABLE, TAKE TWO

The delivery appointment is still on the long side at two to three hours, but it isn't as involved and we're not working directly on the teeth and impacting the soft tissues as much as we did at the prep appointment. About half our patients request sedation again for this appointment and the other half are fine with only local anesthetics. Once the initial discomfort from the procedure goes away after a few days of rest, adjustment, and over-the-counter antiinflammatories, the permanent smile will feel comfortable and natural in your mouth.

REMOVE THE TEMPORARY VENEERS

When the mouth is numb, we'll remove the temporary veneers. This involves making little cuts along the middle of each veneer down to the tooth structure, which allows the temps to come off easily in pieces. With the temps gone, we'll scrape off any leftover glue, clean the prepared teeth, and disinfect everything. Then, with a clean slate, we move to the permanent veneers.

TRYING ON THE PERMANENT VENEERS

With everything set, we'll try on the permanent veneers made by the ceramist. One noteworthy thing about this part of the process if you're getting porcelain veneers: because they have a translucent property, they offer the dentist one more color trick—the shade of light-cured resin cement used to bond the veneer to the tooth. For example, if you think the veneers are just a hair on the darker side and want a little more pop, we can use a bright cement that'll lighten the veneer color a half-step up. On the opposite end, we can use a darker cement to tone down a brighter white to something more natural in color. And we can use a temporary gel the same color as the cement to play with this final tweak to the smile before we do the final seating.

THE FINAL SEAT: INSTALLING THE PERMANENT VENEERS

Once we verify that everything looks and feels good, we're ready to seat the permanent veneers. First, the porcelain veneers are all treated with a hydrofluoric acid etch on the sides that get bonded to the teeth, which creates microporosities on the porcelain's surface. We then place a saline activator on the etched surface, which readies the porcelains to receive a light-cured resin bonding material that gets painted on next. The porcelain veneers are now ready to be bonded to the tooth.

The teeth also need to go through a process to prepare them for bonding. After thoroughly cleaning the surfaces of the teeth, we place a phosphoric acid on the teeth which also creates small microporosities that allow the adhesive resin to flow into those porosities and bond with the ceramic. Like with the temporaries, we'll also add a desensitizer to the tooth surfaces that are getting veneers to help minimize any post-procedure sensitivity. We paint an adhesive resin over the desensitizing material, and now the teeth are ready to be bonded to the porcelain veneers.

We'll use an isolation device, better known as a dental dam, to isolate the bonding site from the rest of the mouth since the bonding process is very sensitive to saliva. We want to make sure everything sticks (quite literally), and that we're not allowing any cross-contamination of the bonding surfaces.

The preselected shade of cement is painted onto the waiting veneers, and they are placed one by one onto the prepared teeth. Then we tack cure the cemented veneers with a curing light, hardening the cement enough to "tack" the veneers in place, similar to tacking a note to a corkboard. The veneers aren't fully bonded to the teeth yet, but the tacking offers us time to go through the whole area and remove any extra cement from around the gums before it's fully set. Then we'll do a final cure on the veneers, which hardens the cement all the way and fully bonds the veneers to the teeth.

With the veneers now permanently in place, we do a final clean-up and check the bite again. As good as our techniques and equipment are for mimicking jaw movements, everyone's joints function a little differently over the course of natural mouth activities. So every time we bond a new restoration on, we must check those jaw movements again to make sure we're maintaining the correct function, and make adjustments. Contrary to what many patients think coming into the process, veneers—and porcelain veneers, in particular—are very adjustable, and they can be repolished and refined in the mouth until they're exactly right. There's a lot we can correct after installation if you close your teeth together and find that something doesn't feel quite right.

Bite checked and with any adjustments made, we give everything a final polish and take one more scan of the new smile to make a second nighttime retainer you'll receive at your follow-up. While the permanents are worlds stronger than the temps, wearing a night retainer is a good preventative habit that protects your new smile from any future clenching or grinding that may occur while sleeping. It also prevents the teeth from shifting over time because, as our patients often hear us say, "Shift happens." Along with other care and maintenance we'll discuss in the next chapter, a retainer can help you get the full lifespan of fifteen to twenty years out of your permanent veneers before they might need to be replaced. With your follow-up appointment booked, you're then free to go and show off your new smile.

PERMANENT VENEER FOLLOW-UP

Before you get too excited about your smile, keep in mind that you'll be seeing us again one to seven days later for a follow-up.

This is a quick thirty-minute appointment in the office, and is similar in purpose to the final blue tape walk-through a contractor does for the owner of a new or remodeled house, which provides a list of fixes for any last-minute flaws.

While we can do other follow-ups virtually, this one should be done in person, as perfecting the bite is tricky, and it can't be checked accurately with photos alone. Similar to the temp follow-up, we like to check the bite after any lingering numbness and swelling goes away and you can feel your bite and tongue the way you normally would. It also takes your mouth time to adjust to the new teeth it now owns, especially since it has just gotten used to the more uncomfortable temporary veneers. While you might be hyperaware of the new restorations at first, and your tongue might play with them a little, that focus will recede as you get used to them.

If, however, there are spots that *don't* recede from your attention, we can address them during this appointment. We'll grind off and smooth out any imperfections and adjust the shape of the veneers to make sure everything about the bite clicks in a good way, and then we'll do a final polish to make everything shine. You'll also receive your permanent nighttime retainer, and we can make some adjustments there for fit and comfort, as well.

The follow-up appointment may be a small step in the context of the whole journey, but it's an important one to help with the longevity of the veneers, as a small bit of rubbing here or there may lead to chipping later. And since function is one of our main goals, we want to send you off with a smile that not only looks good, but also bites and chews the way it's intended to.

Finally, "after" photos will be taken of your new smile, and we'll go over care and maintenance, which we'll discuss in the next chapter.

That's all, folks! Just regular dental cleanings after that.

Oh, and before you ask, you can now go ahead and eat all the apples you want.

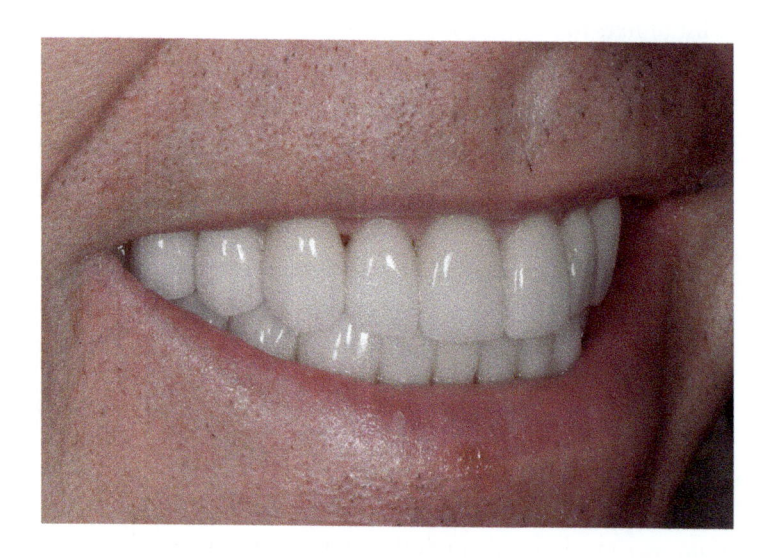

ACCELERATIONS TO THE PROCESS

The normal smile makeover, from your first consultation to permanent smile follow-up, can take about four to six weeks to complete with multiple in-office appointments—about half of that is the clinical process outlined in this chapter. This is a similar time frame to other cosmetic practices. Also expect that it might take at least four to six weeks for popular dentists to get you on their calendar for the consultation.

As you may have guessed from the information we've already shared, several elements factor into the overall timing, including the availability of everyone involved, and the complexity of the restorations. For instance, doing four veneers on the front teeth takes less time to design and execute than a full mouth reconstruction that involves full veneers top and bottom, plus some crowns on the back molars.

For patients whose time is precious, or who are apprehensive about being in temporary veneers for too long because of work commitments or for social reasons, we can speed up the clinical process by using a monolithic material that we can mill and shape in one appointment. However, this means compromising on the aesthetics of the smile, since we can't get the color gradients a ceramist can get using the more time-consuming layered technique done in the lab.

Another factor that can figure into the schedule of appointments is the distance the patient is traveling. We've had people fly in from New York and China, and no matter how dedicated someone is to their smile, they don't want to make four separate long-distance trips out to see us. So, in the spirit of making things more comfortable (because let's face it, travel can be a pain), we can accelerate the process in other ways.

One shortcut is doing all the consultations and model work-ups virtually, including the test drive appointment. Then the patient just has to come in for the two clinical appointments and final follow-up, which we can squeeze into one week. We can still get the pretty aesthetics of lab-created porcelain veneers, which can be made in a week with some preemptive calendar booking with the lab, but this means we compromise on the evaluation process. In these cases, test driving the temporary veneers goes from a week or so to one to two days, which means less opportunity for the patient to assess for flaws and decide on any changes to the smile design, both during and after the delivery of the smile. Though, we will admit, not having the temporaries in for a long time can be a reason in itself for some people to choose to hasten the process, especially if they are sensitive to them. From consultation to delivery, the whole accelerated process takes about three weeks, including the one-week stint in and out of the office.

Because of the compromises that follow time and process accommodations—and the sheer mental and physical demands on our patients—we don't suggest that those who have the means of time and proximity accelerate the process. You will have a better overall experience and feel more confident with the resulting smile when everyone has the assurance all the details are taken care of. A confident process makes for a confident smile.

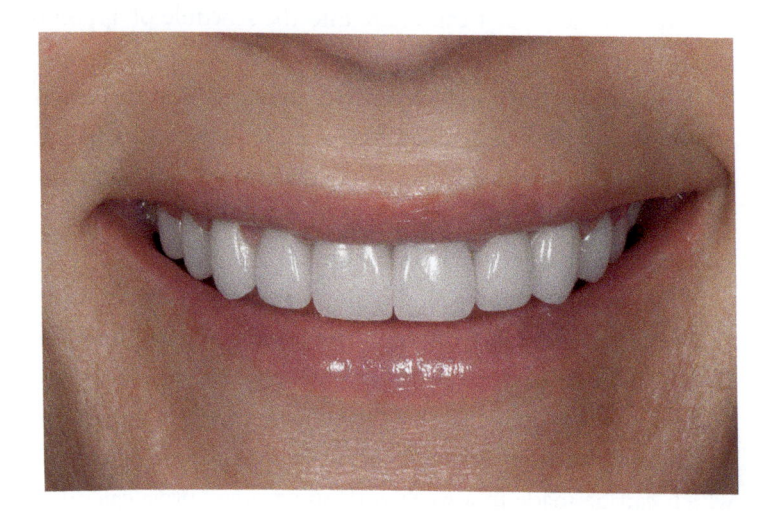

A CONFIDENT SMILE IS WORTH THE WAIT

"There's no way I could adequately articulate how Dr. Field has changed my life," Susan told us, "It's just a smile. Right?"

Susan's smile changed her confidence level. She was inspired to take better care of her health overall, losing weight and eating better. Every time we see her for a check-up, her head is high and her happiness shines through the big smile that now seems to be a permanent feature of her face. She's as happy as can be.

Information is power, and knowing what to expect of the process and what your options are gives you the ability to shape that process and the experience that comes with it. In the end, we want you to be happy, not only with your smile, but also with the experience of getting your smile. Good cosmetic dentists will go over the entire process with you and work with you to get the confident smile you want in a way that's comfortable for you. Because they know getting the smile you've always dreamed about can change your life.

But before you go, there's the question of maintaining your new smile over the course of this life still to address. Prevention is worth a pound of cure, and taking care of this smile investment is your next step.

Chapter 9

Caring for Your Smile

Good oral habits and care are key to maintaining your new smile. If you cheat on your smile, there could be consequences.

One of our veneer patients has an unbreakable addiction to a certain type of chartreuse soda. Even after getting new veneers on his front teeth, he continued to nurse a big bottle of that soda throughout the day, never giving his mouth time to use its natural salivary defenses to buffer his teeth against the drink's acid and sugar. In effect, he created the ideal conditions for a bacterial explosion, which, after a few years, rotted away the teeth that supported his veneers. We had to take off all of his veneers after only three years. We cleaned out the new decay and found we didn't have enough tooth structure left to support a new set of veneers. So, our best choice at that point was transitioning to full crowns.

This all could have been avoided if a little care had been taken with his soda habit. Now, we aren't fans of telling people *what* to eat or drink. We're not dieticians, so we're not qualified to support a person through changing ingrained eating habits. Our recommendations center on *how* to eat—what you can do to mitigate the risk of foods and oral habits—to better maintain your smile.

Once restoration is complete, your new teeth need the same care and attention that natural teeth do. Here are some recommendations for maintaining your new smile to prevent unnecessary appointments and fixes down the line.

BASIC CARE FOR YOUR PERMANENT SMILE, WITH A FEW SURPRISES

Here's the big secret to maintaining your new smile: take care of it like natural teeth. The things we do that damage dentin and enamel are the same things that damage porcelain and polymers. The following suggestions apply to all types of restorative materials, as well as your regular teeth.

BRUSHING

Let's start with the basics: brushing. The minimal recommendation for brushing is two minutes twice a day, after breakfast and before bed. The main objective is to get any lingering food particles off our teeth, particles that feed plaque and decay. This means that, ideally, we should give our teeth a scrub after lunch as well. For people who are more prone to decay, or who have orthodontia that traps food and plaque more readily, brushing after every meal is standard practice. They may brush after snacks as well.

For the average person, any toothbrush will work for this bit of maintenance. However, there are a few specifics. Electric toothbrushes are trendy and effective, and some dentists recommend them over manual toothbrushes. However, if you do use an electric toothbrush, don't scrub with it like you would a manual one. The combination of your hand scrubbing and the electric vibrations can apply too much pressure and friction on your gums, causing harm, like recession. If you go electric, let the toothbrush do its job by running it evenly and lightly over all your teeth as it goes through its cycle of motion.

Variations also exist in manual toothbrushes. If your gums are sensitive or thin and have a risk of recession, soft bristle toothbrushes are commercially available. The softest have a similar texture to foxtail and can gently clean under and around the gum line without causing inflammation. Making even a minor change like this to your daily habit can have compounding effects, such as avoiding a future gum graft.

As for the toothpaste, there are a few general recommendations, and some specifically for porcelain restorations. The advice here isn't that complicated. Over-the-counter fluoride toothpastes like Crest Pro-Health or Colgate work well. If you have some sensitivity, you can use formulations like those found in ProNamel or Sensodyne.

As for the trend of whitening toothpastes, they are fine for regular teeth. As mentioned previously, they don't have much real benefit for whitening teeth, but they won't hurt them. However, it's another story for porcelain. Whitening toothpastes have a high concentration of silica particles—sand, basically—that can scratch and degrade a porcelain veneer's glaze over time. It's like taking sandpaper to a sink. You end up with the opposite of what you wanted, a smile with less luster and a poorer color. There's a consideration for professional polishes used by dentists, too, but we'll get to that a little later in this chapter. The advice here is to check in with your cosmetic dentist on their recommendations for veneer-friendly toothpaste.

FLOSSING

For flossing, the rule is simple: just floss the teeth you want to keep. The minimum recommendation for when and how many times to floss is the same as for brushing, with flossing following brushing. In a perfect world, flossing, like brushing, would happen after every meal since its purpose is the same: to remove food stuck in the teeth and gums.

Floss comes in a variety of nuanced tools, mainly with the purpose of better facilitating its use. The normal floss you get on a spindle in a little box works great, as long as it's unwaxed. If the floss is waxed, it may leave behind tiny wax particles between your teeth and under your gums, which can cause irritation and provide a sticky roost for food and plaque.

If using stringed floss is difficult because of mobility issues, or you have restorative equipment like bridges, temporary veneers, or braces in your mouths that don't allow you to use it properly, there are many types of handheld flossing tools and picks that can work for your situation. Most cosmetic dentists will match you up with the flossing tools that are best for you at any given point in the makeover process. Water picks are also useful in the circumstances mentioned above, and are especially good at removing lodged food from implants. But we don't consider water picks to be a full replacement for thread floss, and the two methods of flossing should always be used in tandem.

RINSING

Here's one big surprise: the way we've always been told to clean our teeth is wrong. Well, not wrong per se, but science says the standard order of brushing and flossing followed by a rinse with mouthwash is not the most effective way to maintain oral health.

The best oral hygiene routine for both natural teeth and restorations is actually to rinse, brush, and then floss.

If you feel like your mind was just blown, that's okay. There is still a lively debate among dentists about this advice, so your own dentist may suggest the traditional way, but here is our reasoning. Starting with a mouthwash rinse does a few things: it flushes out any large pieces of food still in your teeth, stabilizes the pH throughout your mouth, and helps kill or weaken bacteria you can then brush away. This is all accomplished by the alcohol or other antibacterial substance in the mouthwash, but these ingredients are not as good as fluoride at combating bacteria and decay over the long term.

But wait, you say, isn't fluoride one of the main advertised ingredients of mouthwash? To which we say, yes, mouthwash contains fluoride, which helps with sensitivity and acts as a tooth protector against bacteria. It's one of the big reasons people use mouthwashes, to begin with, and the popular reasoning is that you want to do a final rinse with fluoride once the teeth are brushed clean to add this layer of protection, just as your dentist does when they apply fluoride gel after a cleaning. But the fluoride content in over-the-counter mouthwashes is actually a lot *less* than the fluoride content in over-the-counter toothpastes, and definitely less than prescription toothpastes or the fluoride gel your hygienist paints on your cleaned teeth. Rinsing with mouthwash after you brush washes away the stronger fluoride you applied with brushing, replacing it with a weaker dose. Therefore, to keep the stronger fluoride on your teeth, brush *after* you rinse. And once you're done brushing, don't rinse with water, just spit and move on to flossing.

To reassure those who worry about fluoride levels, the amounts found in household products are nowhere near a level that would harm anyone if they are used according to package directions. Know that *not* using fluoride, however, can increase the risk of tooth decay, infection, and sensitivity. For patients who have softer teeth, a lot of gum sensitivity, or a propensity for decay, we recommend toothpastes with higher concentrations of fluoride than normal, sometimes going to prescription strength. But for the normal person, the average over-the-counter toothpaste is enough.

Flossing still comes last because it digs out the stubborn food particles and plaque still hiding between your teeth after rinsing and brushing. It also helps to work any residual fluoride from your toothpaste in between your teeth, where it can remineralize the areas that are most susceptible to decay. Because you want to leave as much fluoride in your mouth as possible for that long-term protection until your next brushing, we don't suggest doing a final rinse after flossing, either. Flossing is your final task, and you can then go about your day. Once you get to nighttime, though, there's another consideration for proper maintenance.

GUARDS AND RETAINERS

Your cosmetic dentist will most likely give you a night guard or retainer to help protect your new veneers. For us, this is standard practice. Or, you may have one to help mitigate general health issues caused by clenching and grinding. If you have a guard or retainer, wear it. It's your insurance policy against a too-soon trip to the dentist to fix a veneer or crown. Unfortunately, your guard or retainer won't help maintain your smile by sitting in your medicine cabinet or in a vanity drawer.

For a quick distinction, a retainer is similar to the clear plastic trays used to straighten teeth. They are thinner and, therefore, more fragile than guards, but work for most people with normal jaw movement. Night guards come in to help with real issues with the temporomandibular joint, or TMJ—the clenching and grinding that we would diagnose early in the smile makeover process because of the tell-tale health issues it leaves behind. Night guards are made of thicker, stronger material designed to better hold up to continued stress and put the jaw into a better position to limit this stress. Guards act more therapeutically to help the jaw, while retainers focus on protecting the new teeth.

Retainers and guards are so important because we generate more force with our bite at night than we do when we're awake since our senses are dulled and the body doesn't have the awareness to stop. Even for people without noticeable parafunctional issues, a lot of unusual jaw movement happens in some dream cycles. Unless we wake up with stiffness or a headache, these movements go unnoticed.

Wearing a retainer or night guard not only helps with protecting the integrity of restorations by reducing their daily dose of friction and stress, but also helps keep them aligned. We fixed the bite during the smile makeover process, maybe we even altered it slightly with the shape of the veneers themselves. But, as we said before, shift happens. We want to prevent bite shifts—and any resulting tooth breakage or crowding—as much as we can.

The biggest patient concern with retainers is comfort. It may feel awkward and bulky at first—it can take up to three weeks to fully acclimate to a retainer or guard—but once your mouth adjusts, it'll feel like a natural part of your daily routine, similar to how your body adjusts to the feel of a new pair of shoes. If you have a digitally designed retainer or guard made by a dentist as part of your care plan, know that these are thinner and more individualized than over-the-counter guards. We also adjust this piece of equipment according to patient feedback when it's tried on in the office, and can adjust it again at a follow-up to make it more comfortable.

In terms of cleaning the guard or retainer—and this applies to the clear trays used to align teeth as well—it's important to brush and soak them every day in denture cleaner or white vinegar to remove any plaque or food that gets rubbed off on them from your teeth. Limiting this cross-contamination is another reason why brushing after every meal or late-night snack is advised. You don't want to be reinserting a guard or tray that traps food or bacteria up against your teeth for hours. That just invites decay and gum disease. For a really deep clean, bring the device to your dentist at regular check-ups where it can be put in a professional cleaner, similar to those used to clean jewelry, which uses ultrasonic vibrations to sanitize every crevice.

CHECK-UPS

Of course, twice-annual check-up appointments and cleanings at a dental clinic are the normal standard of care. This is what's covered by most dental insurances, and constitutes the minimum amount we'd want to see you per year. In addition to a twice-yearly cleaning, the purpose of these regular appointments is to catch and monitor any issues that may come up with your smile before those issues become serious and require more intense intervention. Again, prevention is worth a pound of cure.

Like everything else in the makeover process, this schedule needs to be individualized. For those with higher risk or more complex dental health issues, we want to increase the number of those appointments. For a few patients, that means every other month, which can feel like a lot, but if the choice is between more small check-ups to maintain a smile, and a more intense makeover later to fix a broken one, most people would rather invest in the extra preventative care.

As an added consideration, if you have porcelain veneers, it's important that the practice that does your cleanings knows how to handle them. A lot of the standard dental polishing pastes hygienists use on those little rotating brushes to clean regular teeth can abrad and degrade the glaze on porcelain, shortening their lifespan and impacting their aesthetic properties. Cosmetic dentists use a polishing paste specifically designed for veneers, and that helps maintain their glaze and luster.

Aside from the hygiene component of smile care, there is also a short list of dietary and oral habits we want you to be mindful of. But first, we'll start with the why of caring for your smile.

WHY CARE FOR YOUR NEW SMILE?

You don't buy a new car and then decide not to change the oil, rotate the tires, or speed over curbs. Generally, people want to protect that investment and make sure they get their money's worth before they have to get another car. Since your smile is more important to your personal health and well-being than a car, why should it be any different?

We use our mouths constantly during our waking hours, every single day. Most of us even use them in our sleep. Your teeth do a lot of the heavy lifting of chewing. Since many people hold their tension in their jaws, our teeth can also be mistreated by the daily grind of joints caused by stress. Finally, some use teeth as tools for non-food items—replacements for metal scissors or pliers or vises—which can do a fair amount of damage to enamel and bone. This amount of use means your new smile needs regular care, maintenance, and a few changes of habit to compensate for all of this wear and tear.

When they are well maintained, quality restorations like porcelain veneers and implants can last for up to twenty years. Crowns reach the end of their viability around ten to fifteen years. Ill-maintained, a restoration's lifespan may only be about three to six years. Unlike other industries, dentists don't want repeat customers within a decade. We prefer one-and-done with minimal complications.

When veneers reach the end of their life cycle, one of two things happens. Either individual veneers start to fail and need to be replaced, or multiple issues occur on multiple restorations, signaling that the whole set needs an upgrade. A patient may also decide they want a total refresh as their restorations age out because of changing aesthetic trends. Even for teeth, the ideal whiteness of fifteen years ago is not the "in" color for smiles now.

No matter the cause of the failure, whether it be time, an unsatisfactory first makeover, too much soda, or opening candy wrappers, the result is the same: you have to go through another smile makeover and are responsible for the cost of that in terms of both time and money. Granted, the subsequent makeover process will go quicker, but we'll still have to update records, models, design, and materials, and you'll still have to test drive and go through prep and seating. Therefore, it's in everyone's best interest to be mindful of some general care to get the maximum amount of life from your new smile.

TAKING THE EDGE OFF DAMAGING DIETARY AND ORAL HABITS

Again, anything that can harm regular teeth can also harm restorations. What follows is the lineup of our usual suspects—the dietary and oral habits that cause the most damage to young veneers. Many of these culprits are well-known to people, but some have managed to skirt under the radar of popular listicles and advice.

ACIDIC FOODS

The high acidity found in drinks like soda and coffee demineralizes regular teeth and opens them up to decay and permanent staining. In terms of aesthetics, veneers don't permanently discolor from these drinks like natural teeth do, but veneers can still get a surface build-up that darkens the smile.

The bigger issue with these beverages for veneers, like for normal teeth, is the acidity, but for a different reason. Porcelain doesn't demineralize like enamel, but the acidity can weaken the interface between the porcelain and the tooth itself and shorten the lifespan of the veneer. This type of breakdown is caused, to varying degrees, by all acidic foods. Aside from coffee and soda, some of the other heavy hitters are tea, red wine, and tomatoes. Anything that changes the normal neutral pH in the mouth will accelerate the deterioration of time.

Therefore, for general maintenance, it's important to limit the amount of time these foods and beverages spend in the mouth. If you're drinking a bottle of soda, the worst thing for your smile is to nurse that soda over a couple hours. That doesn't allow your saliva to come in and buffer the effects of the acid before another sip. It's better to get the acid bath out of the way quickly so the mouth can reset its pH faster. Drinking water or brushing after consuming acidic foods can help neutralize pH as well. And, of course, regular check-ups will get your smile scrubbed and polished professionally, remove tough stains, and address any erosion caused by acid.

SUGARY FOODS

The same recommendations given for acidic foods also apply to sugary foods like candy and, of course, the soda mentioned earlier (a double-whammy of acid and sugar). Eating a chocolate bar after lunch is better for your smile than sucking on hard candies all day, which never gives your teeth a chance to recuperate. Sugar, both processed and in its starch form found in snacks like crackers and chips, rings the dinner bell for the plaque and bacteria that cause decay. Like the acid that wears away protective enamel and bonding material, we want to put a short time limit on sugar's stay in the mouth. Brushing or drinking water after treats can help here, as well.

JAWBREAKERS

There's an insidious jawbreaker out there, and we're not just talking about the candy. We're talking about ice, or more specifically, chewing on ice. Regardless of whether it's cubed or crushed, ice is bad. It's bad for regular teeth, veneers, crowns, implants—all types of smiles, really. This is because the structural make-up of ice creates a lot of force when we bite down on it, causing fractures and cracking over time that can pop off veneers and crowns and chip normal teeth. If this makes you think that you should also be cautious with other hard food items like bones, you're right. Chewing on bones can apply the same force as ice and can cause veneers to fracture.

But while ice is bad, the number one killer of veneers is bread. Namely, artisanal bread. You heard us right, that wholesome, innocent-looking crusty sourdough that holds a prime spot on your dinner table is on cosmetic dentists' Most Wanted. Due to their solid structure, regular teeth are capable of munching through that delicious chewy crust with little problem. However, it's another story with veneers because of the way they are bonded to the teeth.

When we eat bread, we bring our lower jaw forward to meet the upper jaw in order to incise it. Tooth edge meets tooth edge in a complex shearing motion that creates a lot of force. That's how we bite into bread. It's an unconscious process, the product of thousands of years of bread-eating. But what happens with a crunchy or chewy bread crust is that when we go edge to edge with our teeth, we put high amounts of pressure on exactly the wrong place for a veneer and they can chip or pop off.

Now, we like a good rustic loaf as much as the next person, so we're not saying to take bakery bread off your table completely. However, to save your veneers, we highly suggest leaning into the idea of "breaking bread" by cutting or tearing chewy bread into smaller pieces that can bypass the front teeth and let the molars take care of chewing. This level of care does not apply for the soft, pre-sliced name-brand breads you get from the grocery store aisle.

As a last piece of advice, there's one more habit unrelated to food that can cause damage to teeth.

TEETH ARE NOT TOOLS

Teeth are not tools. We find that many patients come in with damage to their teeth, both natural and restorations, as a result of using their teeth for something other than chewing food, such as opening packages, biting off clothing tags, or using their mouth as an extra "hand" to hold things in place. Unless you have a disability that prevents their use, hands were made to do those jobs, often with the help of metal tools. Human teeth were made to chew food and smile, and, in order to keep them healthy, those are the only tasks they should be used for. We know it may take an extra minute to find a pair of scissors to open that package, but your smile will thank you for it.

TEMPORARY VENEER CARE

While most of this chapter is about the general care and maintenance of your permanent smile, we do want to add a few notes for the few weeks you manage temporary veneers.

Just like with permanents, you'll want to rinse, brush, and floss—this time with special flossers or water picks—after every meal. As we discussed in Chapter 8, your dentist will go over a recommended care routine at the end of your prep appointment. Also, remember that temporaries are delicate compared to permanent restorations, and are mainly there for looks and feel instead of function. If they can't stand up to eating whole apples, they definitely can't handle killer breads. So, knives and forks are your best friends while you have them in.

Unlike porcelain veneers, it's important not to forget that temporaries are temporary, and made to crack off given the right pressure. To avoid delays in the makeover process, we don't want them to have an excuse to do so until we're ready.

This concludes our list of usual suspects, but we want to make one more plea for taking care of your smile.

TAKE CARE

A little effort and care protects your smile investment and maintains proper health. No matter the age, no one wants to resort to dentures.

Veneers and other restorations are still connected to real teeth and bone structures. Maintaining the veneers means maintaining the health of your entire mouth—bones, gums, jaws, and teeth—because you don't want the biological structures the restorations are rooted on to decay. A restored smile is not a free pass, it needs to be taken care of.

Like everything else about the smile makeover process, your

personal oral hygiene at home needs to be customized to your needs. Nothing, not even your toothbrush, needs to be cookie-cutter. So bring even seemingly minor issues up with your dentist so they can offer appropriate recommendations.

Caring for smiles is not the same for everyone. Health history—which includes genetics, preexisting dental disease, and dietary habits—factors into the best care plan for you.

Drinking soda all day or chewing ice with your new veneers are habits that are probably not worth the consequences if they result in a damaged tooth. If you spend a little time and attention on your smile—and maybe three dollars on a pair of scissors—you'll keep your new pearly whites, and your renewed confidence, for decades to come.

In sum, take care of your veneers just like natural teeth. Rinse, brush, and floss at least twice a day. Go to your annual check-ups. Adjust your habits around high-risk foods. And only use your teeth for eating and smiling. Comply with your dentist's instructions.

While we've given you the best recommendations we can to prevent harm to your new smile, we know mishaps and mistakes do happen. So what do you do if a complication occurs? Let's look at what can go wrong and what to do about it.

Chapter 10

Typical Questions and Complications

After having veneers for about a year, patients usually start to get very comfortable with them. This was the case with Daniel. He got so comfortable, in fact, that he kind of forgot he had them. He stopped treating them as precious, and the care instructions he'd been given (and followed for the first several months) went by the wayside.

When he showed up in the office to address a chip in his one-year-old veneers, we asked what he'd been up to. A bit sheepishly, he replied, "Yeah, remember when you told me teeth are not tools? Well, I was in a meeting, and I opened a candy wrapper with my teeth without thinking about it. It chipped off a piece of my veneer." At least he was honest.

We fixed the veneer. Lucky for him, he was still within our "no questions asked" warranty period, which is *not* standard for most dental practices. If he'd come in five years later, he would have been on the hook for the full cost of repairs.

While we weren't thrilled the patient had damaged his veneer so soon, chips, like shifts, happen—and the best thing to do is know how to fix complications when they arise.

We've now gone through the whole process and talked about some bigger concerns, such as anxiety, that commonly come up as someone goes on their smile makeover journey. We hope most of your concerns have been answered by the previous chapters, but we do want to provide one final clean and polish to make sure we hit all the questions and scenarios that might come up during and after your smile makeover.

This chapter addresses common questions, concerns, and complications that come up during the smile design process and what to expect from a procedure after it's done. These won't be true for all patients, or even most patients, but we thought it important to give them some space here.

The frequently asked patient questions in this chapter encompass the smile makeover process overall and apply to both temporary and permanent veneers. Some of them also address specific procedures we didn't talk about as much, like implants. Much of this information echoes previous chapters, though here we'll keep our answers quick and to the point, and let you know if another chapter will help provide more detail for a particular concern. Finally, we have ordered the questions from what applies to the largest number of patients to what applies to a few.

IS MY MAKEOVER GOING TO HURT?

The short answer to this question is, *not much*.

We talked a lot about comfort options for any potential pain or awkwardness caused during appointments in Chapters 7 and 8, if you need more details, but the basics are as follows. We numb up the mouth and can provide sedation so you feel nothing but some pressure and can relax through the long appointment.

Sedation also reduces any anxiety triggered by the thought of the procedure itself. Other than its length, this procedure shouldn't feel too much different than a normal cleaning.

As for aftercare, there should just be some inflammation and sensitivity for a few days, and maybe a little more achiness in the jaw if deep decay or old restorations had to be removed during the prep appointment. These discomforts are typically managed well with over-the-counter ibuprofen. There will also be some hot and cold sensitivity because of the plastic of the temporaries themselves.

For permanent veneers, of course, there shouldn't be any discomfort after installation. Take a couple ibuprofen until the immediate inflammation recedes a few days later, and that's it.

As for other procedures, such as the sensitivity caused by whitening agents, we use appropriate comfort measures there as well. Desensitizing material and fluoride treatments are common solutions for this.

WHAT DO SMILE MAKEOVERS COST?

In 2023, the cost for veneers and crowns ranges anywhere from $1,500 to $4,000 per tooth. For whitening, you're looking at $500 to $1,000 for the whole mouth, depending on whether you're doing it at home or in the office. For us, implants will be $3,000 to $7,000 per tooth, but we can do our implants within the practice. For other dentists that partner regularly with other professionals, the cost could be higher. These ranges account for the training and skill of the dentist, lab costs for labor and materials, and the complexity of the patient's case. For instance, an implant that calls for a bone graft will cost more than one that doesn't, as it will involve an oral surgeon who has their own fees. Market conditions in your area will also factor in.

While dental insurance will cover some of these costs if the restoration is related to health, say a crown for a cracked tooth or replacement of a broken down restoration, insurance doesn't prioritize aesthetics, or even the longevity, of a restoration. Dental insurance, in our humble opinion, is a sham. It's not really complete insurance, but a defined benefit under a healthcare insurance plan, and typically covers up to $1,500 to $2,500 a year on any dental work. This number equates to your six-month cleanings and maybe a crown. We explain how it works to our patients with this inelegant comparison: If your car gets hit by a rock, you pay your deductible, and your car insurance covers the rest. If your head gets hit by a rock, you pay your deductible, and your health insurance covers the rest. If your mouth gets hit by a rock, your dental insurance will pay the maximum they allow, which is around that $2,000 mark, and you pay for the rest.

One thing you can do to help supplement your regular dental insurance is add a health savings account (HSA) or flexible savings account (FSA) to your health insurance plan. These are often offered as options through employer-provided benefits. These savings accounts put pre-tax dollars from your paycheck into an account that can be used for medical or dental bills not covered by your insurance plan. Be sure to read the fine print, as there are different ways HSAs ask for proof a payment was made for medical reasons before they will approve a transaction. Another common supplement for dental costs is third-party financing programs. You can think of these as credit cards for dental work.

The big lesson on cost: be prepared to pay for cosmetic restorations through means other than your dental insurance. We don't think putting the onus on patients is fair when it comes to long-term health and confidence, but it's the healthcare system we have for now, and good dentists do their best to work with people to help them plan and budget for a makeover. For instance, some dentists may offer payment plans or split payments for longer, more involved makeovers.

HOW LONG DO SMILE MAKEOVERS TAKE TO COMPLETE?

There's some variation in the timeline, depending on if you're getting a smile upgrade or a full smile makeover. As always, the schedule will vary depending on the needs of the individual, but the approximate times for procedures are:

- Whitening—If it's in the office, it takes about an hour and a half. At home, it takes a daily application over the course of seven to ten days to get the desired effect. Note that whitening does not last forever. Depending on eating habits (i.e., if foods that stain are a major part of the diet) the procedure may need to be repeated in one to three months. Whitening is a little like the Botox of the dental world.
- Porcelain veneers—In total, it takes four to six weeks to complete the veneer process, from initial consultation to permanent installation. The two main clinical appointments that prep, test drive the temporary veneers, and seat the permanent veneers use up one to three weeks of that total.
- Crowns—Depending on the materials and where they are placed in the mouth, crowns are a one- to three-week process.
- Implants—Because an implant often involves other oral professionals and some additional steps, healing after the screws are implanted, it can take a while to deliver the final implant. Implants clock in as the longest restoration at three to nine months. If they involve complex orthodontia, it will take even longer.

If orthodontics are involved in any smile makeover, the makeover process will automatically be extended to provide the time necessary for the teeth to be aligned correctly. In our practice, we can do orthodontics that use graduated clear plastic trays, which slowly move the teeth into shape. For orthodontia that requires changes within the jaw, like correcting an overbite or to move a tooth to close a gap, braces and bands come into play. These bigger shifts can take months, sometimes over a year.

There are a few accelerations to the process of tooth alignment, such as devices that use vibrations, or a technique called micro osseous perforations, in which tiny perforations are made in the bone along the tooth roots to create a cellular response that moves the teeth faster. The combination of these techniques can cut the time of orthodontics in half, but you're still looking at a few months at the least.

When it comes down to it, the best way to keep within a decent time window is to be on the ball and comply with your orthodontist's or dentist's instructions. There's no benefit to us if the process is delayed—in fact, the frustration caused for everyone by an extended process is decidedly *un*beneficial—so we'll always give you the best-case timeline and tell you exactly how to meet it.

HOW DO YOU CARE FOR TEMPORARY VENEERS?

Here's a quick summary of Chapters 8 and 9 on how to treat temporary veneers because of their weaker materials and construction.

Temporaries stain more readily than porcelain or real teeth, so watch out for food with strong colors, like coffee, red wine, tomato sauce, and turmeric. You may see a difference in coloration from beginning to end, even in the short amount of time you wear them.

Temporaries fracture more easily. It's part of their nature, since they'll soon be removed. So take care with your eating habits while they're in. No biting into hard or chewy foods. Cut up main meals into smaller bites and let your back teeth do the work of eating.

WHAT HAPPENS IF THE TEMPORARIES BREAK?

It's not a huge problem if the temporaries do fracture during their three-week test drive period. We can fix them in the office quickly and easily. The biggest issue with a breakage is the inconvenience of having to come in again before the seat appointment.

HOW LONG DO PERMANENT VENEERS LAST?

As stated in Chapter 9, well-maintained permanent veneers can last between fifteen and twenty years. After that, we either start replacing individual failing veneers or do an entire smile update by replacing the old veneers with new ones. Because materials and techniques are always progressing, the updated set will look and function better than the old.

WHAT HAPPENS IF MY VENEERS DISCOLOR?

Related to longevity, patients often ask us if porcelain veneers discolor. The short answer is no, but those heavily pigmented foods can lay down a top layer of stain that at-home brushing may be unable to remove. However, an office cleaning with a porcelain polish will clean them right up.

Polymer material, being plastic, will discolor over time, a known issue your dentist will help you plan for. Zirconium restorations are too opaque to discolor. And if your veneers get dulled from inappropriate toothpastes your cosmetic dentist can polish out the scratches to restore their glossy finish.

The other thing that can happen is the teeth underneath the veneers can darken over time, which causes the translucent veneers to darken as well. If this happens, we can use a whitening product to lighten the back of the teeth, or replace the veneers.

WHAT HAPPENS IF I CHIP MY VENEER?

If a veneer gets chipped for whatever reason, the obvious next step is to call your dentist and make an appointment to get it fixed. Small chips can often be smoothed and polished during a quick office visit without compromising the aesthetics and strength of the remaining veneer. Larger chips can sometimes be repaired, but usually require the individual veneer to be replaced. Again, since permanent veneers are not connected to each other like bridges or temporaries, if one is damaged, only that one needs to be fixed or replaced.

WHAT HAPPENS IF MY VENEER POPS OFF?

If the veneer comes off altogether, start by finding and preserving the veneer. If it's whole and clean, chances are your dentist can rebond it to its tooth with minimal fuss. Even a broken piece may be saveable. The exact container you store the veneer in doesn't matter, as long as it's clean, sealable, and food-safe (this is something that will go back in your mouth, after all). We've had patients come in with veneers wrapped in paper towels, empty prescription bottles, and Tupperware. Any container that's easy to see and handle, and that has a tight seal will reduce the chance of the veneer being lost or broken more in transit.

Once you've secured the detached veneer, follow the same steps as with a chip and call your dentist. We'll clean and sterilize the veneer, take off the old bonding material and apply fresh cement, and do our best to reattach it. Once bonded back onto the tooth, we'll polish it up so you won't be able to tell it came off.

For veneers damaged to the point where they can't be replaced—or if the veneer was reaching the end of its lifespan—we'll replace it with a new one that matches.

WHAT IF I NEED A ROOT CANAL?

Teeth that start the smile makeover process with a lot of preexisting decay or disease might be at risk for future nerve death of the tooth root. We do our best to catch these issues with scans and X-rays before installing the new smile. Since we always prefer going with the most minimal intervention, if the decay is close but the nerve is still healthy, we can remove the decay using a technique called a pulp cap. Pulp is the dental term for the nerve inside the tooth, and the cap refers to a seal that's placed over the top of the nerve area that protects it from infection and stimulates healing around the nerve. Effectively, the technique heads off a root canal.

In cases where a root canal cannot be avoided, such as true nerve death, we partner with an endodontist to do the necessary root canal. If the tooth with the root canal is included in the smile design, it will often get an individual crown instead of a veneer, which will be made to match the rest of the smile.

However, there are rare borderline cases where a root canal is needed after the permanent smile is installed. This happens when we don't see the need for a root canal before the makeover because the decay isn't yet adjacent to the nerve, but biological quirks caused by stress from the procedure can progress the problem faster or further than we anticipate. In these cases, a skilled endodontist can do the root canal around the veneer, preserving the new smile.

WHAT ARE THE SPECIAL COMPLICATIONS OF IMPLANTS?

Because they're a more complex makeover than veneers and include surgery, implants have a few potential complications that veneers don't, mostly related to the surgery that implants the screws into the jaw bone. These include the normal list of post-operative risks for any type of surgery that impacts bone, such as bleeding, swelling, infection, and lack of integration (a.k.a., the bone doesn't fuse to the implant). It can also include potential issues indicated during consultations with the various professionals involved. For instance, if a patient never grew an adult tooth, the bone at the site of the missing tooth may be insufficient to anchor an implant, in which case an oral surgeon will do a bone graft to provide that anchor point, or insert a special anchor that acts in a similar fashion to a drywall anchor.

For run-of-the-mill post-op bleeding and swelling, time and acetaminophen will help. Remember, because ibuprofen impacts bone healing, it is *not* recommended for procedures that involve the jaw bones.

If infection occurs, depending on its extent and how quickly it's found, local and systemic antibiotics may be able to treat it. In more intensive implant surgeries that require bone grafts, there's also a higher risk of infection around the implant site in the bone itself. This requires removing the implanted material and letting the healing process start over, a delay that doesn't usually impact the smile's end result.

As to the rarest complication, we typically test for bone integration a few months after the jaw heals around the implanted screw. If the screw is not completely fused to the bone, we remove it, regraft the bone, let the new bone heal, and come back to place a new implant. Usually, we experience no further problems after the second attempt. However, if there's a preexisting biological reason for the rejection, like a metal allergy, we'd have to move to plan B, usually a different surgical procedure or a bridge. As shown in previous chapters, complete rejection is rare because we can catch a majority of potential issues like metal sensitivities early on and adjust the smile design and materials to compensate.

This completes our list of frequently asked questions. You may have others unique to your own situation, which your dentist can answer during any point in the makeover process. It never hurts to ask. And we encourage you to ask questions even if they sound silly. It can't be sillier than, "Can I eat bread?," and that certainly has a more interesting answer than anyone expects.

COMPLICATIONS HAPPEN

Understanding what complications can occur helps minimize the risk of them happening, and having a dentist that has this knowledge to share makes the smile makeover process less stressful and more successful. But sometimes, there's little anyone can do to foresee and prevent a complication, and all we can do is recover from it.

"I appreciate all your hard work and patience dealing with such an impossible and challenging case like mine, Doc!" a former patient recently told us. "Can't wait to see you again!"

His parting words took us aback a little, since he'd experienced many ups and downs to get to his new smile. This is when you know your team is doing something right because "can't wait to see you again" is not a sentiment dental offices are known for inspiring.

Working with someone you trust to competently and correctly make things right is often an overlooked part of good aftercare. Complications happen. They are a part of life, and your smile is no different. There are thousands of ways that a smile can be impacted, from the serious to the silly. No matter what was at fault for the complication—be it human error, mechanical failures, or biological variance—in the end, it just needs to be worked around or fixed.

Now that you know what to expect when you're expecting a new smile, you're ready to live your life with the smile that reflects the best of you.

Conclusion

LIVING THE DREAM SMILE

Procedures and practical advice now shared, we bring it back to the beginning of this whole makeover journey.

What makes you smile?

For Joanne, it was surviving melanoma. "I didn't know if I was going to live or die," she says in a video testimonial of her makeover experience. "As long as I have my health, there isn't anything I can't do. I'm alive. I feel blessed."

Joanne's case was unique. She'd just beaten cancer. So, with a renewed feeling of purpose and optimism, she wanted to count the blessings she still had. One of those blessings was the opportunity to fix a broken tooth she'd been putting off. After facing down cancer, the dentist's office didn't seem so daunting anymore.

But the issues with her smile went beyond a broken tooth. An untreated bite issue had caused a lot of wear, and now both her teeth and her ability to chew were compromised. That's why she'd broken a tooth; the system was not functioning correctly.

Because of this, she was looking at a long line of minor fixes for chipped and broken teeth through the rest of her life.

We gave her two options. Through door number one, we could keep fixing her teeth, one at a time, as they broke. And through door number two, we could look at her entire smile holistically and do a full smile makeover, starting with correcting her bite, then getting the teeth positioned the way they needed to be, and finally, making those teeth look better.

After the valley of shadow she'd passed through, it's no wonder that Joanne loved the idea of creating a new, confident smile for herself. "Let's do it!" she said.

And we did. We collaborated with Joanne through the entire smile design process, from using digital images to see exactly how her new smile would look on her own face and adjusting details until the design was right, to a smile test drive with a mock version of her new veneers so she could see the physical smile, to the permanent porcelain veneers that light up her face and make her look as blessed as she feels. She's thrilled. Every time she comes into the practice for her regular dental check-up, she can't help but share her smile. She says the biggest compliment she gets from friends is, "That smile is so much more *you*."

"What's not to like?" Joanne says, giving a big, slightly tearful grin, "It's a dream come true."

Joanne's fear of the unknown was overcome by the anticipation of getting her dream smile. New beginnings are rare. As a central part of the face and the primary communicator of emotion, the smile can be the biggest little makeover of a person's life. It's not so much that other people will see a confident smile (although they will) but that *you* will feel and know you are confident.

Joanne's experience was more dramatic than most, but the smile makeover process she went through at our office was not. A smile really is a new beginning. And it's not just the new smile that should give you confidence, but the dentist and the makeover process that help create it. A good cosmetic dentist will walk you through the smile design process from start to finish, helping you create, plan, and test drive your new smile so you know exactly what you want, how much it will cost, and what to expect at each step of the process and beyond. In short, a good dentist will treat people, not teeth.

Because of our early training, dentists can fall into the role of technician or tooth mechanic, with treating disease as our only goal. We don't think about how to treat the person, and can get wrapped up in what we think will look and function the best. Therefore, it's important that you establish a relationship with your dentist and dental care team and clearly communicate what your expectations and desires are. Not just what you want your smile to look like, but what you want your smile to *accomplish*. That way, you can form a working partnership that will zero in on your ideal smile design and foster trust that your dentist can do what it takes to get a smile you will be happy with.

Tooth structure is not a replaceable commodity. While the degree of skill and patient collaboration may differ among dentists, as a species, we genuinely want you to have healthy, functional teeth that look good. Some of us are better at delivering on those outcomes than others. If you are interested in pursuing a smile makeover, we encourage you to reach out to us and other cosmetic dentists for a consultation. Many cosmetic dentists even offer virtual consultations. Talking to a dentist doesn't mean you need to commit to anything, but it will give you the information you need to make an informed decision. And we encourage you to shop around and do multiple consultations to find the practice that resonates with you.

Though we've outlined the average trajectory and stages of the smile makeover for the average person, we want to emphasize that this process can be adjusted in infinite ways to make it right for you. A smile doesn't come from a recipe or brochure. It's not made with a cookie cutter. This means it's crucial to work with a knowledgeable, experienced, and well-trained dentist who knows all of the options from A to Z that can and need to be done to ensure you go into the process feeling confident. To get your confident smile, you need to be confident in the makeover process that gets you there.

Restorative technology has progressed, and keeps progressing, since the dreaded days of the hyperreal Chiclet smile. Now, strong, functional, and beautiful porcelain veneers can give you a smile that looks and feels like the real thing, with minimal impact on healthy tooth structure. Smile test drives can translate your vision to your own facial features, creating the ideal smile just right for you. And sedation options can help limit any stress or discomfort that may come with longer prep and seat procedures. Finally, you now know the latest recommendations for care and maintenance and how to handle common issues, which will help your smile look great far into the future.

A smile makeover is a process. If you try to rush it, you may not get the results you want, and there's no do-over for a smile makeover once tooth structure has been altered. Take the time to do it once, and do it right, by trusting and fully engaging in the process. Every step of the makeover process, from design to care, is subjective. In other words, the exact details of the process must be customized to the individual. Your fears, artistic preferences, health history and needs, lifestyle habits—down to the bread you eat—make or break the success of your smile makeover.

And now we'll end where we began: with the importance of the smile. Socially, it says a lot about who we are and what we value. We are judged by our smiles before we even get to speak, which can considerably alter someone's prospects when a first impression counts, such as in the case of interviews and first dates. Once a person has achieved the smile they've always wanted, the confidence of knowing those first impressions will be good ones lifts the stress of social encounters.

We've seen countless personal transformations like Joanne's at our practice. Renewed confidence lifts a person's whole bearing so much that they are hardly recognizable as the same person when they return for a check-up. But they are the same person—just, more so. To paraphrase Joanne's friends' responses to her smile, the restored smile seems to make people more themselves. As if the person they are inside finally becomes visible on the outside, and a new happiness comes from the freedom to fully express themselves and communicate with others on their terms. That happiness spills over onto everyone else. That's the real reason smiles light up a room.

A new smile can be life-changing to someone's feelings of confidence and self-worth, as Joanne, Sarah, Mary, and many of our other patients have found. Yet, even after they have their new smile, so often we hear people express feelings of guilt about spending money on themselves. We think the shame of perceived selfishness is partly why some patients hide the fact that they've had work done to fix their teeth. No matter who or what else pulls on your priorities, time, and budget, it's important that you know this: *you are worth a smile that makes you want to smile.* You are worth a smile that makes you healthier. That makes you feel more confident. That makes you want to lift your head high when you walk into a room.

You are worth a smile that makes you look more like *you.*

It's okay to invest in all of that. It's okay to make a change for the better. It's okay to want to smile again. A car does much less for us personally, yet we don't think twice about making that kind of investment.

The importance of the smile is not just tied to aesthetics, but to overall health. Neglecting your smile doesn't make problems go away, it only makes them worse. Proactively giving your smile the attention it deserves according to its level of personal, social, and medical importance is key to getting not only a confident smile, but also a long-lasting and durable smile that works with as much of your natural teeth and bone as possible. Don't wait. Be proactive about addressing smile concerns early to avoid bigger restorations later.

The smile design process is a journey you don't want to miss. It's an exciting adventure into self-improvement, and taking it slow to understand and make contributions to that improvement can lift a person's mental confidence as permanently as their smile lifts their physical confidence.

Your smile matters. You don't have to continue through life feeling like a movie villain. You don't deserve a broken smile that makes you feel like anything less than your best. Teeth get heavy use as the chewing machines they are, and genetics, time, and other priorities coalesce into a perfect storm of smile breakdown. Teeth don't heal like other injuries. The scars on them don't fade. But you don't have to be ashamed of a life lived: you can choose to invest in your own health and confidence and get the smile makeover you've always wanted.

It's your smile—show it how much you care. And live life confidently.

Acknowledgments

The reality is that we all stand on the shoulders of giants. There are many incredible doctors who came before me and changed hundreds of thousands of smiles. I am so grateful for those with an abundance mindset who have shared their experience and knowledge with me and given me an opportunity to build on their foundations. From my time at USC, to the thousands of hours of continuing education, I've been blessed to have great mentors and teachers who shared so freely with me. I pray that through this book, I can pay that forward and help others understand how important our smiles are, and that we live in a time where we can help anyone create a smile they are confident with. I would also like to acknowledge my ceramist, Daniel Sorenson. I've been able to work with him my entire career, and the reality is, I couldn't do the work I do without him. Lastly, thank you to those who helped me make this book a reality—from my coaches and mentors at Fortune50, to the team at Scribe Media, and to my patients, who are my inspiration.

About the Author

Called the "go-to cosmetic dentist in the San Francisco Bay Area" by local media, DR. JOSEPH FIELD dedicates his practice to improving the patient experience. He was first exposed to dentistry by Operation Smile dentists while on a service mission to Colombia. There he saw lives changed for the better through modern dental practices and came home intent on helping to do the same.

He earned his DDS from the University of Southern California's famed dental school—where he also learned to love college football and hate LA traffic—and was credentialed in implant reconstruction and smile makeovers. A key thought leader in the field of cosmetic and reconstruction dentistry, Dr. Field is a Fellow in the Academy of General Dentistry (FAGD), a Fellow in the International Congress of Oral Implantologists (FICOI), a Fellow in the American Academy of Implant Dentistry (FAAID), and a diplomat for the American Board of Oral Implantology (DABOI). Passionate about sharing his knowledge with potential patients as well as industry colleagues, he has over thirty articles published in publicly accessible sources, including *WebMD*, *Well*

+ *Good*, *NBC News*, *HuffPost*, *Business Insider*, Medium's *Authority Magazine*, *NewBeauty*, and *Reader's Digest*.

When he's not restoring smiles, Dr. Field likes experimenting in the Peninsula Center for Cosmetic Dentistry's ceramics lab and coaching his fellow doctors and team members on improving patient care. Outside his practice, he also teaches at his alma mater, and lectures around the country on advanced techniques in cosmetic and reconstructive dentistry. He lives with his wife and four children in Los Altos, California.

Find out more about Dr. Field, his partner dentists, and the Peninsula Center for Cosmetic Dentistry at https://pccdsmiles.com/.

www.ingramcontent.com/pod-product-compliance
Ingram Content Group UK Ltd.
Pitfield, Milton Keynes, MK11 3LW, UK
UKHW020843200225
455344UK00009B/51/J